Parkinson's Warrior

Parkinson's Warrior

By Nick Pernisco

Published by Connected Neurosciences LLC

Connected Neurosciences LLC
1037 NE 65th St. #80832
Seattle, WA 98115

www.ParkinsonsWarrior.com
info@parkinsonswarrior.com

Ordering Information:

Quantity sales. Special discounts are available on quantity purchases by corporations, associations, and others. For details, contact the publisher at the address above.

Orders by U.S. trade bookstores and wholesalers. Please contact Ingram Book Company: Tel: (800) 937-8200; Email: customerservice@ingrambook.com.

Printed in the United States of America

Cover design by Marianna Bernshteyn

Ebook: ISBN 9780578418292
Print: ISBN 9780578418230

First Edition

10 9 8 7 6 5 4 3 2 1

Parkinson's Warrior is dedicated
to my wife, Rosaline Bernstein,
and to my mother, Teresa Pernisco.

Preface

First things first - I'm not a doctor nor a lawyer, I don't pretend to be a doctor or a lawyer, and I don't play one on TV (or YouTube). What I *am* is a well-informed, engaged Person with Parkinson's (PWP). My intent is to provide you with information and inspiration to help guide you through your Parkinson's journey. While you will learn all about Parkinson's, and you will be able to speak the "lingo" intelligently with your doctors, your family, and your friends, this is not a medical book, per se. This is one Person with Parkinson's reaching out to hold the hand of another Person with Parkinson's.

Always seek your doctor's advice and follow their instructions before starting any new medication, beginning any exercise routine, or changing anything about your routine. In these pages, you will find interesting ideas, both scientifically proven and anecdotal, that you may want to go out and try right away. My advice is to first talk about each new idea with your medical team and get their input before deciding on a change. My hope is that you will find out about new therapy ideas, learn the basics about how these therapies work, research them further on your own, then be informed enough to have a true discussion with your team – one in which there is a back and forth of ideas, not one which your doctor says "take this and call me in a month." A good doctor will always welcome your input, and a great doctor will admit when they don't know enough about a topic and will be open to continue learning.

Acknowledgements

This book could not have been written without the help of so many people. To everyone in the Seattle Parkinson's community – Nate, Suzanna, Dr. Witt, Stephen, Tim, Tom, Kent, Sally & Patty, Ken, Veronica, and to everyone else a part of the PNW PD family – thank you for your inspiration. To my colleagues at SMC – Nancy, Brad, Maria, Sara, Sharyn, as well as Mitra, Peter, Matt, Kevin, Fran – thank you for believing in my ability to continue my work after diagnosis. Thank you to my friends and family for their constant companionship and support, with strong ties that cross a continent and an ocean – this book was written because of your love.

Introduction

There are at least one million people diagnosed with Parkinson's disease in the United States, and up to 10 million around the world. This means that, including loved ones, there are more or less 100 million people affected by this disease worldwide. You may be one of these people.

Perhaps you have just received a diagnosis, or perhaps you have known for years. Perhaps your husband or wife has been diagnosed with Parkinson's, or perhaps it was your father, grandfather, mother, grandmother, son, or daughter. Perhaps you are a friend of someone who has just been diagnosed. This is a disease in which the more you know, the better you'll live your life. Understanding how those of us with Parkinson's should take care of ourselves, how to fight the daily battles, and how to develop a long-term plan for living well will help us lead better lives. This book will provide those of us affected with the tools we need to take control of the illness and improve our lives.

When I was first diagnosed, I went through a long spell of depression and uncertainty. Before Parkinson's, I thought I had my life figured out, but everything I was working toward went out the window after receiving the diagnosis bombshell. I felt like my life was over and I was emotionally lost. Faced with the prospect of having a shorter amount of time to work in my career, to do everything on my "bucket list,", or even worse, of becoming disabled before I could do anything more with my life, I frantically jumped into every new thing at which I thought I could succeed. I thought I had to have new experiences and check off all of the items on my bucket list before it was too late. I tried going back to school several times, I started a new company, I ran for public office, and I did many more zany things. I overwhelmed myself, and I eventually burned out. That was when I decided I needed to change how I approached the treatment of my disease, but more importantly, how I approached life. I wasn't the same person before being diagnosed, and things needed to change if I wanted to be happy and as heathy as possible.

I learned everything I could about Parkinson's, and became an expert patient. I read all of the books about Parkinson's, both for patients and for professionals in the field. I read all of the latest research and began keeping track of all of the new treatment options. After a few months, I knew more than enough to have an intelligent and productive discussion with my medical team. I could work with them, for example when they would suggest a new medication, and we would be able to have a lively debate during our appointments. I learned all about medications, supplements, exercise, nutrition, and everything else related to the disease and its progression. I developed my own system for tracking the various aspects of the disease, and eventually developed a mobile app that made it easy for me to keep track of the various aspects of the illness.

In addition to information, I believe all PWPs need some inspiration in their lives. Life with Parkinson's doesn't need to be about living life with negative feelings. There are ways to live a happy life while also living with Parkinson's. My hope is that my story will serve as an inspiration to you and that my experiences can help guide you and make life a little easier. Parkinson's is a very difficult disease to deal with, but it's not an impossibly insurmountable mountain. Besides the motor symptoms we experience, we also could have cognitive and emotional difficulties to deal with. It's possible to strengthen our minds and overcome these emotional obstacles. There's currently no cure for Parkinson's, but you can still live a full, happy life.

While I'll talk about improving your health through exercise, diet, and by finding emotional well-being, I'll take you down the road of my own struggles with Parkinson's, and how I refused to let it keep me down. I won't pull any punches – I plan to share all of the information you need to know; the good, the bad, and the ugly. In the end, my hope is that you will be able to understand what is happening to your body, and you won't fall for misinformation and tacky sales tactics frequently found online. You'll learn that there is hope, and that there are reasons to be optimistic – it's worth repeating over and over: you can live a happy and full life with Parkinson's. I taught myself to fight, to become a Parkinson's Warrior, and I'll show you how to be one too.

I'll talk about how at first, I refused to accept that I had this disease, and how this led to a lot of heartache. Once I admitted it to myself, that *I was sick*, I was able to move forward and redefine what I wanted my life to be about. I'll also share some thoughts that I've come to realize as truths about life, and along the way perhaps you may discover some truths about your life as well.

When you're done reading this book, you'll have a general idea of what Parkinson's is, how it's treated by mainstream and alternative medicine, and about developments being made to help improve the lives of PWPs and to find a cure. You'll find that I refuse to sugarcoat anything. Medications can have some terrible side effects, and the late stages of Parkinson's aren't pretty, but I'll talk about them alongside all of the gains that can be made by understanding them. I'll talk about how people die with this disease, and how you can improve your chances of living longer and preventing an early death. Let me make this clear: nobody with Parkinson's HAS to die prematurely. There are ways to protect yourself and to increase your chances for a long life. I was diagnosed at age 33, and I plan to live until at least 80! You can too.

My hope is that this book motivates you to take control of your health and to fight like you are battling a fierce enemy – because you are! When Parkinson's was first identified as a disease, it was labeled the *Shaking Palsy*. I call Parkinson's the *Ballsy Palsy* – it tries to win the war every single day of our lives. It thinks it has the upper hand and that it will defeat us. But we can combat it, first with information and then with action. Information is useless without action, and action is useless without first understanding what is necessary to win. The ancient Chinese strategist, *Sun Tsu*, said "Every battle is won or lost before it's ever fought." This is especially true with Parkinson's disease. It's important to have a strategy for how to fight each battle so that we may live a full and healthy life. Don't worry, you'll have an entire army of people behind you – your doctors, your family, your friends, and other PWPs you meet. Remember, information is power. The more you know, the more options you have in your life.

I invite you to reach out to me if you have any questions, suggestions, concerns, or just need some guidance. I'm happy to connect you with any resources that might be helpful (hint: start with the appendix at the end of the book!).

Nick Pernisco
nick@parkinsonswarrior.com
http://ParkinsonsWarrior.com

Table of Contents

Chapter I

My Parkinson's Story

It's worth beginning our journey by going back in time and telling you my own Parkinson's story. If you have just recently been diagnosed, you'll be able to relate to the torrent of emotions I experienced when I was first diagnosed. If you have been living with the disease for a while and you're struggling, my hope is that you will find some peace in knowing that you are not alone in your struggle. There are people who understand you and what you're going through.

The First Symptoms

Like most people eventually diagnosed with Parkinson's, you may have discovered a small change – the appearance of a minor tremor in a finger, a tightened arm muscle, people telling you that you look sad – and you thought nothing of it or just wrote it off as normal aging. For me, it was the tightening in of my left arm. My left arm felt like it was extremely tight and I couldn't relax it. It felt like the arm was in an invisible sling and was just stuck. Since this symptom appeared in what seemed like from one day to the next, I thought it was just some inflammation from playing tennis. I visited my general practitioner and he concurred with my assumption. He prescribed 800mg of Ibuprofen, several times per day, for six months. I was satisfied that this would resolve the issue and went on my merry way.

In retrospect, I had other symptoms before the stiff arm, but I ignored them, thinking they were only temporary and would go away on their own. About a year before the arm, I had begun struggling with a bit of depression for no particular reason. As it turns out, depression is a known Parkinson's symptom, likely caused by the lack of dopamine going through the brain. At around the time the arm became stiff, I took a fall on the tennis court and sprained my left ankle. I had also been experiencing more fatigue and could not play tennis for longer than an hour. All of these things taken individually do not mean much, but to a trained eye, these symptoms are the beginnings of a neurological disorder. Stiffness, slow movement, a dragging foot, depression, fatigue – all signs were clearly aiming towards Parkinson's, but it would still be a while until I was anywhere close to a diagnosis.

After the six months of Ibuprofen, and with no improvement whatsoever, my doctor decided to escalate the examination by sending me to a senior doctor. By now, some friends were suggesting I see a neurologist, but since my health plan was with an HMO (Health Maintenance Organization – a bureaucratic healthcare system with all of your medical needs centrally coordinated), I had to go through this awful process of seeing many more tiers of doctors before seeing a movement disorder specialist or having any kind of specialized tests. The senior doctor examined my arm and the rest of my body. By now, my left foot was dragging (likely what caused the fall and sprained ankle), and I had begun having stiffness in my left hand. He said neurological problems like these don't affect 31-year olds. He also thought it was some sort of inflammation, but since I insisted on seeing a neurologist, he eventually conceded.

Apparently, my HMO only had two neurologists on staff in the Los Angeles area, despite being the largest health organization in that metropolitan area. This meant that I had a two-month wait for an appointment to see a neurologist. The first appointment was where I first learned that there was a possibility that this was Parkinson's disease. I knew nothing about this disease and only knew that Michael J. Fox had it, and watching what he had gone through, I was more than just a little scared. I was shocked. My first question to the neurologists was, "Is this fatal?" His answer was a little disconcerting, saying that "anything can kill me," but that he wasn't sure yet so let's not get ahead of ourselves. Not very comforting! He wanted his colleague to confirm, so I waited another two months for the next appointment with the other staff neurologist. This second neurologist concurred with the first, but they still couldn't believe someone so young could have Parkinson's. However, they thought there was enough probability that I should see the movement disorder specialist.

The movement disorder specialist (THE, because there was only one in all of Los Angeles), was an older man who had recently retired but who was seeing patients occasionally on Tuesdays and Thursdays. If I was diagnosed, this person would oversee my care – for how long, I wasn't sure. This doctor saw me walk into his office, and after speaking with me for about a minute, he said he was almost sure it was Parkinson's. To confirm, he gave me a one-week regimen of Sinemet (also called carbidopa-levodopa). If my symptoms improved while taking carbidopa-levodopa, I had Parkinson's. I took the carbidopa-levodopa for a week, and could honestly not tell the difference between being medicated and unmedicated.

This was when the doctor was determined to find out once and for all by choosing the nuclear option – quite literally!

A PET (Positron Emission Tomography) scan is different than a CT or MRI scan in that it's supposed to show how the brain works. It does this by using radioactive tracers to map out the various routes in the brain. There is a definite brain pattern for someone with Parkinson's, and this test would show whether my brain was consistent with that pattern. I had to wait nearly four months for this test, because the radioactive tracer needed to be harvested, and there was only one facility in Southern California that could do it, and they were behind schedule in their production. But eventually the doctors had the material and called me in for the scan. I had an early-morning appointment, since I had to be fasting for the test. Before the test, I was given some pills containing the radioactive tracers, and a little bit of water to wash them down.

About an hour later, I was led to a very cold, dark room with the big PET scanner in the middle. I was prepped and the techs helped me get my head into the machine. I was strapped down so my head couldn't move – moving my head would have been bad, apparently. The techs left the room and shut the door, and the machine came to life. I laid there quietly for about 30 minutes as the scanner did its work. My thoughts raced, and my fear and anxiety were muted only temporarily every five minutes as a tech would ask over a loudspeaker if I was ok. I wasn't ok.

At the end, I was given a card that said that I was radioactive and would be for 24 hours. I was supposed to show this card to anyone around me so they would know I was dangerous to be around. Later when I got home, I turned out the lights, but to my dismay, I did not glow in the dark.

Diagnosis

"You have Parkinson's."

These three little words confirmed our fears on a cold December evening in 2011. All of these doctors were baffled for nearly two years trying to pin down a diagnosis that just didn't quite fit into their academic or professional experiences. "The patient is young, never did drugs, never smoked, rarely drank, otherwise completely healthy, and with no family connection to this disease." It made no sense. It still makes no sense.

As a practical matter, the movement disorder specialist decided to give me the news by email through the hospital's messaging system. "Your test result is consistent with that of a person with Parkinson's, so from now on we will treat you as such. With everything this could have been, you're lucky you have Parkinson's." I stood up from the computer and walked to the bathroom mirror. I studied my face for a moment – I already exhibited the "masked" expression that PWPs often have, with my left eye appearing to droop slightly – and I began thinking about how my life would now change forever.

I knew it could have been worse. It could have been ALS, MS, or any number of other horrible acronyms. I could have ended up in a wheelchair in a year. I could have been a horrible burden for my family. The eternal optimist thought for a moment, "Thank God, Parkinson's."

Facing the Music

In life, we know that nothing is certain, that things can change in an instance. We try to ignore the little voice in our heads that tells us, "you're going to die one day." We need to ignore it. Thinking about death all of the time is no way to live. But we get constant reminders, almost daily. We watch the evening news and see the death around us – a crane falling on a car and killing the driver, a mother shot while she was taking her daughter to daycare, a pedestrian struck by a drunk driver. We listen for the details and try to learn our lessons. "Oh, that happened in so and so neighborhood. I never go there," or "That was a freak accident. What are the chances?" We convince ourselves that bad things will never happen to us.

When I was younger, I'd see people in wheelchairs or walking funny with a cane, and my parents would say "Don't stare!" I'd still stare, but find a way to do it when they couldn't see me doing it. "What happened to that person," I thought. "Were they born that way? And why can't I stare?" As I got older, not staring turned into looking away, almost ignoring. I didn't want to be caught looking at someone else's disability. I'd imagine it might be embarrassing enough for them. I knew that I'd be embarrassed to walk like that. But I knew that couldn't happen to me. "Whatever that person has is probably due to some freak accident. What are the chances?"

Until it happened to me.

I was the person starting to show signs of illness. My left arm continued to stiffen, to the point where I'd just avoid using my left arm for anything. My left foot began to drag behind me. My voice became very quiet. Typing was starting to get very difficult. I was afraid, and I mean really afraid, for the first time in my life. I had always been very introspective, but I became even more so after my diagnosis. How would this disease progress? How many years would I have left to be productive? Could I die from this? Would I be one of those people my parents told me not to stare at? Why was this happening to me?

It's no wonder that I began feeling depressed and filled with anxiety. There were so many uncertainties. Everyone with this disease progresses differently, so I didn't know whether I'd be at the end stages in five years or forty. It's been said that the only constant in life is change, but this was way too much for me to handle. After all, everything that I had known about my life – how I'd wanted my career to progress, the vacations my wife Rosaline and I would take each year, and even where we'd end up living – it was all up in the air, never to return to the ground in an orderly fashion.

Shortly after my diagnosis, I began having really horrible and vivid dreams at night. Even though I was raised Catholic, I had never considered myself to be a person of faith. This didn't change after my diagnosis, but these dreams made me feel different about the world around me. In several of the dreams, I was floating above and outside of my own body. I began seeing myself, not as someone with control over his own life, but rather as a small piece of a greater whole – a tiny ant in a huge ant farm, a small cog in a huge system, an 80-year life in a sea of billions of other 80-year lives. I saw a future with earth as a barren, lifeless wasteland. For the first time in my life I had to face the fact that one day I was going to die, and my dreams were playing this out by showing me just how small and insignificant I really was.

These were very sobering thoughts for a 33-year old who was previously happy and healthy. At the same time, these thoughts were very liberating. Although the intervening years from then until now would bring a lot of heartache, and at times I'd forget about the lessons from these dreams, it was at that time, and with those dreams, that I had discovered the meaning of life.

But I'll come back to that.

At the time the dreams were occurring, almost nightly, my depression and anxiety were only increasing. I couldn't stop thinking that I'd no longer have the life I'd hoped for. I had done a lot of good things in my life, but I had never done anything really great. Now that I was facing my eventual disability, I felt even more sorrow for the fact that I had never pushed myself to do more. Now, I thought, it was too late. If you think that I was being whiney and melodramatic, you'd be right. But all I could think was, how could this happen to a smart middle-class kid who rarely drank, never smoked or did any drugs, and who was caring and thoughtful. Looking back now, I realize, why not? I'm only human. This could have happened to anyone. But at the time, I just couldn't accept it.

I began my long, arduous journey through the five phases of grief. While the psychology of grief and loss has been well studied and documented, its effects and the duration of each phase vary by individual. For example, my own way of dealing with the five phases – denial, anger, bargaining, depression, and acceptance – was to spend the first few months in denial. I would just go about my business as usual and I would ignore that anything was ever wrong. During this time, I thought I was going through the five phases very quickly, and I thought I had reached acceptance in month three. At the time I thought, "Ok, I have Parkinson's. This isn't too bad. It should be easy enough to keep doing my thing." Looking back now, it took several years to finally find acceptance, which is what has allowed me to finally tell my story. Those several years were filled with a combination of denial, anger, bargaining, and depression – often all at the same time.

I knew that, even though I couldn't accept what was happening to me, I had to tell my friends and family. Rosaline was with me at every doctor's appointment, so of course she knew everything. Everyone else had to have known something was wrong, but what? I had to tell them, right? I thought it would break my mother's heart. Maybe she didn't have to know. I could go for years without her knowing anything was wrong. But I have never kept anything so serious from my family. I'd tell my family, even though it would be extremely difficult. But first, I'd practice by telling my friends.

We all have people we're close to; friends, family, friends you consider family. After years of knowing each other, the group had become very tight knit, and almost very homogenous. Most of my friends at the time were long-time friends I had met in college. We all liked the same kind of movies, the same kind of restaurants, used the same laundry detergent. None of my friends were known for sticking out, for being too different. This is what made me really afraid to tell them. I was afraid of sticking out. Would our relationship change if they knew? Of course it would, but all relationships change over time. I'm sure they had noticed that I had perhaps lost a skip in my step, or that I was not as animated and gregarious as when they first met me. All of us would get old, and we'd all invariably get some chronic illness one day. I'd just be the first.

I first told my closest friends. They suspected that something was wrong because of the stiffness in my arm, and I had kept them up to date with what was going on. First it was my friend Mathew. We went to a local bar for someone's campaign event – one of Mathew's neighbors was running for city council. We were both interested in local politics and were excited to meet some local leaders. Also, they were buying the drinks, so we said 'why not?' After a couple of Margaritas each, I broke the news.

"So remember I had that neurologist appointment last week? Well, it turns out the arm thing is Parkinson's."

He reacted with a gasp and I explained a bit more.

"I'm not going to die, but it's going to get worse."

We talked about it for a few minutes, and then I changed the subject. It was tough letting someone in on my secret, but I felt a huge sense of relief afterwards. Now that the first one was done, maybe the next ones would be easier. I developed a sort of shtick that I'd repeat with different friends. I'd get alone with each person – going on a walk up in the hills above Culver City or going to dinner at a favorite restaurant. I'd work it into the conversation somehow and repeated the performance over and over.

"I have Parkinson's. I'm not going to die, but it's going to get worse."

After about a month of my diagnosis, my closest friends all knew. The most awkward moment was when I told my friend Guy over the phone. He lived in Seattle and there was no other way to tell him unless we went for a visit, which we did a couple of months later. Rosaline thought I should have waited to tell him in person, but I wanted him to know. After mentioning it, the conversation got quiet and I ended it before it got too awkward. Later that night, I got a text from Guy:

"You know I'll always be there for you."

The sentiment was shared by all of my friends, but seeing it on my phone like that made me appreciate it even more.

Over time I've put a lot of thought into why it was so difficult to tell people about my diagnosis. Most people keep diagnoses like these secret due to their job – it's too easy for an employer to put you on the chopping block first during layoffs or when something goes wrong. It's understandable – most bosses don't want to deal with an employee who will produce less and require special help. This is especially true in corporate life. Since I began my journey I have met several people with young-onset Parkinson's who were let go from their jobs within months of disclosing their diagnosis. As a professor, I worked for a government agency and had union protections, so I wasn't too worried about getting laid off.

The reason it was so difficult to tell people I had Parkinson's was because I thought others would see me as weak, and they would begin thinking of me as that person in a wheelchair from my childhood. I could already imagine myself in my wheelchair and people averting their eyes as I rolled by. Like too many other times in my life, I was more concerned with how others would view me than anything else. I was, of course, being overly dramatic. I had just been diagnosed with a progressive illness and I couldn't help but to take my mind to the extreme. Later I'd discover that I was only partially right about this.

The hardest part was telling my family. I knew that I had to tell my mother first. I had never kept serious things from her – yes, I could be considered a mama's boy – and she would find out soon enough anyway when my symptoms worsened. I'd rather I broke the news to her in a controlled setting rather than have her imagine the worst and then get upset because she didn't know. I planned to tell her the next time I was over for dinner, since that happened frequently enough.

It was a dark winter afternoon as I was heading to my mother's house for dinner. At least once a week I'd have dinner with her and chat for a while, then go home and take Rosaline a plate of hot homemade food, which she always appreciated after getting home late from work.

That day I got there a little early, while the food was still about half an hour from being ready. We always tended to eat on the earlier side, at around five thirty or six, since the pasta was pretty heavy and it wasn't best to eat so much before going to bed. The television was always on loudly, mainly for background noise, usually tuned to a Spanish-language channel. I turned the television off and called my mother over to the sofa and told her I needed to talk.

I said that I had gotten some news from the doctor about my arm. I explained that it wasn't just some inflammation and that it was something I'd need to deal with, but that it wasn't too horrible – I always tried to downplay the severity of anything serious when I talked to my mother.

"The doctor says it's a disease called Parkinson's."

I went on to explain how the disease worked, what effect it would have on my body, and critically, that it isn't fatal. I could still live a long life, but things would just be more difficult for me going forward. Even though I tried to be gentle about it, she still got upset. After I finished, she said her stomach hurt and she rushed to the bathroom and locked herself in there for ten minutes. I stirred the pasta sauce until she came out, and I could see the devastation on her face. This was the reaction that I feared.

Parents are supposed to worry – that's part of the job description. There was a lot of uncertainty at the time, but I did my best to allay her fears. I explained that the worst was still decades away, though I knew the worst could be just around the corner.

Over the next few weeks I told some other family members, while I knew the news would trickle down to others. I told my brother and sister and they immediately began offering up advice. "Don't stress," "take it easy at work," "don't push yourself," etc. Rosaline told her family, so that helped me avoid an awkward conversation with my in-laws. Her dad's response was classic – both representative of his personality and true to the reality: "Well, life goes on."

Life did go on.

I can't fully describe the level of support I received from Rosaline during the turmoil and aftermath of finding a diagnosis. She was there at every doctor's appointment, and she provided a rational voice that balanced out everything going on in my head. Just five years into our marriage, we both understood that I could soon become a burden rather than an equal contributor to our household and participant in our lifestyle. She has been the strong one on many occasions since.

Despite Rosaline's support, I began to worry about our future. Some PWPs I had spoken to suggested I consider early retirement. My condition would only worsen, but I could stave off progression if my main priority in life was my health instead of earning a paycheck. Being 33 years old, this sounded like a ridiculous notion. I was hitting my stride in my career. I was well respected at the college, spoke at conferences around the state, and was getting more involved in local politics. I had no plan of slowing down or stopping any of this. But reality would soon smack me right in the face.

The Downward Spiral

In 2010, I was teaching at Santa Monica College, and had also been actively involved in college politics. All of my classes were scheduled on Tuesdays and Thursdays, and after a while I had developed a routine. My day consisted of waking up at 6:00am, shaving, showering, having breakfast, and driving 15 minutes to school. Each day I'd be sure to arrive at 7:00am to check e-mail, drink my coffee, and meet with students. I began teaching at 8:00am, and taught until about 3:30pm. I worked this schedule twice a week for about seven years.

My teaching schedule gave me the opportunity to explore other interests, such as starting and managing a small business. When the iPhone was released in 2007, I knew I wanted to be involved in this digital revolution, so in 2009 I launched a company selling ringtone apps – not the most consequential of businesses, but we can't all be Apple or Microsoft. I used my background in digital audio and radio to record actors saying things like "You've got a new Facebook message," and you could set these as custom alerts on your smartphone. I released this on Blackberry, Android, and iPhone, and the business quickly took off.

I had originally learned that my illness might be Parkinson's in mid-2010. Rosaline and I grieved the situation, but were still hopeful. We would not let this get our lives severely off track, but that doesn't mean that we didn't plan for the worst-case scenario. We began saving more money each month, spending less on eating out and on frivolous trinkets. We made sure that our medical insurance was appropriate to handle a severe illness. I knew that there would be a time soon when I'd not be able to teach in the classroom anymore. I didn't know when that would be, so I had already started asking if I could teach from home through the school's online system. We didn't know what to expect with this disease, so Rosaline also began looking into future career options.

Rosaline's was ready for the next step in her career, and we would prioritize stability, since if I had to take early retirement and could no longer work full time, we could possibly not survive on her income alone. If we wanted to future-proof our family, we would need to make a drastic change. Luckily, I had married a dreamer, albeit one whose feet were more solidly on the ground than my own, so we put our imaginations to work.

What can someone do to survive when their life is about to be turned upside down? Our unlikely solution was to go with the flow and embrace the coming life revolution. I vividly remember the moment we would decide our future. Rosaline and I were trying to come up with ideas for how to move forward. What would be the best way to ensure at least one of us had a stable income going forward? The unlikely solution was for her to close her company and go to business school.

Ever since I could remember from a very young age, I was surrounded by business. My parents ran their own business, my cousin was very successful with franchises, and even family members in other countries had their own businesses. We are an enterprising family. In school, I had considered studying business, but decided at the time that the math requirements were just too much. Rosaline had no problems with math, testing into Calculus in 10th grade. We had a conversation about business schools, and how many students who enter are her age and go on to have stable careers at large multinationals. A quick look at the UCLA MBA and discussion with some friends who were MBAs confirmed this. It appeared as though companies were fighting each other over hiring even those at the bottom of their class. I suppose if you graduate from UCLA, you have met a minimum standard, since they are very selective in their admissions process. Even those at the bottom of the class at a top MBA program are likely to be extremely high achievers.

Rosaline knew that to have one of these successful careers, she would need to go to the top school. In Los Angeles, UCLA and USC were among the best. It would be expensive, costing around $100,000 to attend. But we saw it as a way to help our family in the long run. It was an investment in our future. But there was still much to think about and do before a final decision could be made. Could we survive for two years on my online teaching salary alone? We had our families to help us emotionally, but financially we would be on our own. This is where the dreaming came into play.

"We have friends in the northwest. What if we moved to Seattle," she asked me. After all, she argued, rents were less expensive at the time, and our cost of living would go way down. Since I had already asked to teach from home in future semesters instead of going into the classroom, this idea of moving and keeping my job was actually plausible. The difficulty came in the fact that our lives were already being turned upside down, what would happen if we left the place and the people we were so familiar with for something new and unknown? At first, it seemed like a great idea, a new adventure and a new reason to dream about the future. Little did we know what was in store for us.

While making an effort to support Rosaline, I had my own demons to battle. Moving away from my family was indeed very tough, and leaving my classroom teaching job and business, combined with my new diagnosis, really spiraled me into deep depression. I just could not come to terms with all these changes happening at once in my life. In my first couple years in Seattle, I must've seen four or five different therapists about these issues. There was a lot on my mind.

I kept thinking, how long will it take for this to get worse? What does my future hold in terms of my career and my life with my family and friends? I had a few friends in Seattle, but would be able to make new friends? Would people notice my illness, think there's something weird about me, or not want to be my friend because of it? I went from being a happy, optimistic person who loved people, to being someone who just wanted to be inside and forget the world. I remembered how my parents told me not to stare at the person in a wheelchair or showing a disability, but now I was the one showing the disability. I experienced the fears that I only imagined up to that point – fears of being rejected, fears of people staring at me, and being embarrassed when I'd try eating a hamburger or burrito and making a mess of it all. It's the fear of being different.

The best way I knew of to get past this stage of my life was to find something to focus on and with which to move forward. After a year of Rosaline being in her MBA program at the University of Washington, I got it into my mind that I wanted to be in the program as well. It would be a great way to form a new community and learn skills that would serve me well in the future. I was also feeling so down on myself that I needed external validation – some objective indicator that proved I was still valuable to society. I had never been good at math, so I took math classes to help my chances of getting into business school. I was hoping my new math skills along with the fact that I had previously launched a software company would have been enough to pass their selection process, but I was mistaken.

I had read on several message boards for people with disabilities that disclosing your disability was not necessary when applying to a job or to school. I decided to not mention my Parkinson's in my school application, and tried to get in based on my merits alone. I made it to the last phase of the application process – the group interview phase – and was rejected. I was told that, while I looked good on paper, in person I looked awkward and disinterested. This was before I began taking Parkinson's medications, so I had very slow movements and exhibited the "masked face" that many of us PWPs often do.

I was crushed by what had happened. I contacted the admissions office and explained the situation, telling them everything about my Parkinson's and asking them to reconsider. They refused.

This turned out to be a watershed moment for me. If I didn't tell people what was wrong with me, they would assume the worst and they would not see me for who I really was. If I was open about it, I wouldn't need to explain myself and people would just understand, "yes, there is something wrong, but please focus on what's inside." This is when I decided that I'd be open with my illness with everyone I met, and not hide my illness like it was a scary skeleton in my closet. This has garnered mixed results over time, but I certainly think that it was the best thing for me to do.

The next year, I applied to business school again, still disappointed about the previous year's rejection. Not only did I want to prove to myself that I was still capable of this, but I wanted to prove it to the world, especially to the school. This time I prominently featured my struggle with Parkinson's in all of my admissions essays, and I discussed my limitations with the program staff throughout the process. This time I got in. I eventually attended business school and stayed for three quarters, roughly about a year of a three-year program, due to a sudden worsening of stress-related symptoms. I was very involved in school activities, and well-liked by my classmates, who elected me to be first-year class representative. The entire experience had been a sort of vindication for the fact that I had been rejected the first time. During my time back in school, I made the most of the opportunity. I learned a lot, met a lot of great people, started a non-profit benefitting girls in Ghana, and laid the foundation for future endeavors. In the end, unfortunately, my body gave out on me and I could not continue for as much as I wanted to. It was a huge disappointment, perhaps the biggest in my life besides being diagnosed with Parkinson's. After so much success in my life, I thought maybe this was the turning point – everything I undertook from now on would end in failure. After dropping out, many classmates tried to keep in touch me, but I was so embarrassed that I just retreated back into depression.

The Turning Point

It's only when you hit rock bottom that you can begin your ascent.

After leaving business school, I tried a few other things to make myself feel whole, but nothing worked. I was searching for external validation that I was still a valuable human. I couldn't see that I needed to stop with the constant sense of panic that time was running out – time was running out and I was wasting it on trivial preoccupations that ultimately didn't matter. I needed to focus on my health.

In 2016, after nearly five years of being diagnosed, I finally accepted the fact that I had Parkinson's.

By this time, Rosaline was out of school and working. The pressure was finally off of me to care for the family financially. I could focus on improving my mental and physical health. I took a holistic approach, and was determined to learn anything and everything related to Parkinson's. I read every book and article I could find and became an expert on this illness that I might have for the rest of my life. I learned all about medications and supplements. I learned about the best exercises for Parkinson's, and about stress relievers like meditation. Suddenly I was the most knowledgeable person at my support groups. I had a lot of information to share on new therapies and could answer almost any question about Parkinson's.

The cloud started to lift and I felt healthier every day. The positivity in my personality returned, and I began to feel hopeful about the future. So what changed? I'd argue that it was my mindset that was different. I decided to accept that I have an illness that limits me. I also felt useful again, sharing what I knew with others made me feel like myself again – I had a new sense of purpose. I not only accepted that I had Parkinson's, but also that the best use of my time was in trying to live a good life, not in trying to achieve for the sake of accomplishment.

Life should not be spent dwelling on what you don't have, but instead appreciating what you do have. I had a loving wife, a loving family, and loving friends. I didn't need to go to school or get to know a whole new group of people; I already possessed every skill I needed to succeed in life and I was already surrounded by the best people to share my life with. Instead of worrying about the future, I wanted to focus on making the most of the present. I learned that life is not about worrying about the future that may never come, or about things in the past that have already happened and can't be changed, but about enjoying the present moment. I decided to refocus my life on the things I love – spending time with family and friends, traveling, teaching online, writing, and playing pinball.

Since I came to these realizations, I've been able to make changes that have made my life a lot better. My depression and anxiety are well-managed and are no longer a daily hindrance. Although my motor symptoms have progressed, I feel healthier and stronger than when I was first diagnosed. I realized that happiness is not a state of bliss that is all flowers and kittens, but rather it's a choice you make every day and it requires effort on your part. Each day is different, and some days are better than others, but the key is being active and present in your own life. This mindfulness is what makes for a Parkinson's Warrior.

To reach a higher plane of self-love and self-acceptance after everything I put myself and my family through, I feel a responsibility for sharing everything I know for the benefit of others in the Parkinson's community. Hopefully my story resonates with you, and you can perhaps recognize some of my experiences in your own life. It's possible to live a healthy and happy life with Parkinson's, and I'm the absolute proof of that.

Chapter II

What Is Parkinson's, Anyway?

While there had been indicators pointing to Parkinson's as a diagnosis, I waited until being diagnosed to learn much about the disease besides whether it's fatal (it's not). Reading disease information on medical websites always made me anxious, especially since many sites are filled with misleading or otherwise incorrect information. After being diagnosed I spoke to my doctors for more information, but much of what they offered was advice and information about worst-case scenarios. I learned a lot of things that scared me, but knowledge is power and the more we know the better we can battle with it.

Parkinson's disease is a neurological condition that affects how the body controls muscle movement. It stems from the brain losing its ability to create dopamine, as the dopamine cells in the brain either die or go dormant (depending on who you ask). Dopamine is the necessary chemical our brains need to control muscles, but it also affects mood, memory, and so much more. Without dopamine in the bloodstream and going to the right places in the brain, the body slows down and eventually comes to a stop. The best analogy I can think of is that of a wind-up clock – at first the clock keeps perfect time, but as the winding becomes undone, the clock slows down until it finally stops. This is what happens to the body when it loses dopamine. In Parkinson's, this slowness and stiffness in the muscles is called bradykinesia. It's often accompanied by a tremor, as well as psychological and emotional symptoms.

The Ballsy Palsy

Parkinson's was first documented by English surgeon, James Parkinson, in his 1817 work entitled An Essay on the Shaking Palsy. A palsy is defined as paralysis, often accompanied by tremor. 200 years after that seminal work, I'm going to give Parkinson's a different description – the Ballsy Palsy. Parkinson's is ballsy because it acts confidently when it attacks, causing all sorts of mayhem – physical, emotional, and psychological. It affects everyone differently, and each day is a different battle with different symptomatic severities. The disease believes it can take over your life by taking over your body, and perhaps in the past it did. However, today we know how to fight back, and just like fighting back against any arrogant bully, it's well worth the challenge to put it in its place.

No other non-fatal disease sets out so boldly to torture its victims, which is what makes Parkinson's so rough on those of us inflicted by it. It traps you in your body, unable to move, as if you were tied up and gagged in an old Western. The only thing is, the sheriff isn't coming to the rescue. Instead, you are left to free yourself, to find your own way to escape or at least learn to live your life in captivity. But here's the good news: it's possible to fight back against this bully. You are not destined to a life in which you are tied up and gagged, shaking with fear or tremors. We will learn how to fight back, and we will learn from others who have blazed the trail to our benefit.

You may know something about Parkinson's already if you've heard the stories of Mohammed Ali and Michael J Fox. The effects of Parkinson's on each of their bodies are very different. Mohammed Ali's movement was an example of bradykinesia. He moved very slowly, he had a tremor in his hands, his face lacked movement and looked like a mask, and he could barely walk. This is the effect of the body in later stages of Parkinson's and usually manifests itself because dopamine replacement medication loses its effect on the body. Michael J Fox's movements, on the other hand, demonstrate the opposite effect. The dopamine replacement medications – usually a mixture of levodopa and carbidopa most commonly known as Sinemet – have an over-medicating effect that causes the opposite of bradykinesia called dyskinesia. People with dyskinesia have excessive and uncontrollable body movements, usually in the head, shoulders, hands, and legs. These symptoms typically appear after the PWP has been taking the medications for a few years, and occurs when the brain receives too much medication too quickly. I think of dyskinesia as having the polar opposite effect of Parkinson's; when a PWP is dyskinetic, tremor, slowness, and rigidity disappear but they are replaced by these unwanted movements. While there are medications to help tamper down dyskinesia, the movements are almost impossible to stop until the medications wear off. Like with any medication, Parkinson's medications are prescribed to strike a balance between reducing symptoms and causing side effects. Even so, I and many other PWPs often prefer the movement that being properly medicated allows, even with these often-unsettling movements.

The manifestation of Parkinson's in someone's body can happen slowly and over time. When Parkinson's symptoms begin to appear, the brain has already lost the use of 80% of the dopamine cells in the brain. It's typical that someone has been slowing down for years but just thought that it was a part of the normal aging process, until a major symptom like strong tremor or a stiff arm made them go to the doctor to get it examined. Although my first reported symptom of Parkinson's was stiffness in my left arm, I actually had non-motor symptoms years earlier that could have been a hint of more to come. About four years before I was diagnosed, I came down with a serious bout of depression for no reason. Two years later, my arm got stuck in a position against my chest almost as if it was being held up by a sling. The arm is what made me go to the doctor and later to the neurologist, not the depression. It turned out that the depression was probably the first symptom, and that the stress I had experienced made the next symptom reveal itself. Depression is a common first symptom among PWPs, especially for young onset Parkinson's patients.

When most people think of Parkinson's disease, they perhaps think about a grandparent that was afflicted with it later in their life. It's common to associate Parkinson's disease with older people because most of those afflicted with the disease are over 60. However, young-onset Parkinson's disease is possible – I have even met someone with something called juvenile Parkinson's disease, as she was in her teens when she was diagnosed. Young-onset Parkinson's disease is typically assigned to anyone who is diagnosed between the ages of 30 and 50. Young-onset Parkinson's is so rare, that doctors typically initially disqualify any notion that it's even Parkinson's. My own doctors spent two years trying to figure it out, and even after the PET scan, they said Parkinson's was the likely diagnosis. Since I was 33 at the time and I had no family history of Parkinson's, for too long doctors refused to believe there was anything too out of the ordinary. It turned out that without a genetic connection to Parkinson's – genetic testing has ruled out dysfunction in any of the genes currently associated with Parkinson's – and with no exposure to pesticides or having suffered any concussions or major head trauma in my life, my Parkinson's was ruled as idiopathic, having sprung spontaneously and for no known cause or reason. About 10 million people worldwide have been diagnosed with Parkinson's, about a million of those with young onset Parkinson's, and fewer than that with Parkinson's that's idiopathic. It turns out that I'm among the lucky 0.00003% of the world population that will get young onset Parkinson's for no apparent reason. Statistically, I'm more likely to be struck by lightning twice and win the lottery than to get this disease. I'd almost prefer the lightning.

Parkinson's is a progressive disease that gets worse over time, and there's currently no cure for it. There are plenty of medications to help mask the symptoms, and when taken properly in the early stages, many people are surprised at how well they help mask these symptoms. Earlier in my own disease, people I had met after having been diagnosed said that they had no idea of my illness until I had mentioned it – when my meds were working properly, my body language seemed almost normal. But those who had known me for a long time could tell I was different than before I was diagnosed. As time has gone on, the intensity of my symptoms has increased along with the dosage of my medications, and my symptoms have become very noticeable to everyone. And while there is nothing that can stop the progression, there is one scientifically proven way to help slow it down – exercise. Yoga, tai chi, weights, and cycling have all been proven to slow the disease. Some doctors advocate for the use of nutritional supplements to help protect remaining dopamine cells (antioxidants like Vitamin C and Resveratrol are common), and while some supplements do show great promise, and some I'd even consider vital for a PWP, I've found that exercise is the best medicine.

Parkinson's progresses as dopamine cells in the brain continue to die or go dormant. This increases the intensity of the symptoms. Each person experiences the disease differently – Parkinson's is sometimes called a boutique disease – custom made just for each person. The common symptoms are muscle stiffness and slow movements, but many people also experience tremors, loss of balance, depression, and memory loss, as well as some less common symptoms like dandruff, circulation problems, fatigue, constipation, and alcohol intolerance. If I were to not take any medications for two days, I'd wake up very stiff in general, but my left arm and leg would be especially immobile, my body would move very slowly, and my mind would be very cloudy. This is why it's considered a medical emergency if a PWP forgets their pills at home while on vacation or if pills get stolen or destroyed. Often these meds are taken several times each day, and missing a dose can lead to a total body takeover with the full force of the disease.

Though Parkinson's symptoms can be cruel and even agonizing in later stages, people don't die from Parkinson's, but rather from complications like Pneumonia or by taking a nasty fall and breaking their hip or hitting their head. Although it won't kill me, I'm completely aware that the disease could eventually leave me disabled in a wheelchair and in need of 24-hour care later in life if no cure is discovered. Although I'm hopeful a cure or a disease-altering treatment will be available in my lifetime, I also need to deal with the present-day reality – the unpredictability of Parkinson's from day to day has already limited my ability to work full time. Sometimes my body needs to be in bed all day, and sometimes I can do a few household and work-from-home activities, but I usually can't get by without a daily nap sometime in the afternoon. It's also difficult to predict at what times the medications will work correctly and at what times my body just won't want to comply with modern medicine.

Although most studies about Parkinson's involve older people who were diagnosed in their 60s or 70s and involve deaths within 10 years of diagnosis, there is research that shows that people with young onset Parkinson's can reach old age like everyone else. I also know many people who were diagnosed with young-onset Parkinson's 20-25 years ago and who are still going strong and living life, albeit with plenty of modifications and help from others. Two of these people are now in their 60s and still go for walks and take vacations. Although symptoms get worse over time and medications lose their efficacy over the years, there are some options to help improve quality of life in the later stages of the disease.

One procedure is called Deep Brain Stimulation, or DBS. This is brain surgery in which doctors implant a sort of pacemaker for your brain, causing a short circuit that confuses and blocks the disease. People for whom the main dopamine-replacement drug, carbidopa-levodopa, used to work well but has lost its efficacy would benefit from this procedure. People who undergo the DBS procedure often notice a huge increase in mobility and a steep decrease in the intensity of motor symptoms. And although DBS could reverse symptoms and make the PWP feel like they had felt a decade ago, ultimately even this trick loses its efficacy over time – remember, all of the current treatments are like bandages on a disease that keeps progressing.

When someone is first diagnosed with Parkinson's, the first question that they ask their doctor is, "Am I going to die?" Well, yes, we all are going to die. However, the biggest myth I've heard about Parkinson's is that it kills you – that people die from Parkinson's. This isn't exactly true. PWPs die WITH Parkinson's, not FROM Parkinson's. The disease affects your muscles, but your organs remain untouched. Your heart keeps beating normally, your lungs do their thing automatically, as does your liver and other organs. When I read obituaries about people who have died with Parkinson's, I always read through to find out what really killed them. The most common way PWPs die is through complications like taking a big fall because they lost their balance, or by getting pneumonia and not treating it in time. There are ways to prevent falls, and being vigilant about pneumonia and getting proper and expedient treatment will extend your life. I once met an older lady with Parkinson's who later died of Cancer. Unfortunately, having Parkinson's doesn't mean you can't get other illnesses, so living a healthy life is especially important for us.

Of course, just because I can live a long life it doesn't mean that each day will be great. The intensity of symptoms varies day-to-day (and sometimes even hour to hour), and as the medications begin to lose their efficacy, and perhaps even the deep brain stimulation begins to have a lesser effect than when it was first installed, the real struggle begins. This is the time that most people feel that they are entering the phase of disability. I've seen people in this late stage of Parkinson's, and it isn't pretty. People in wheelchairs, crouched over, drooling on themselves – and I can only imagine the psychological and emotional effects as well. It's terrible to think that this is the future for many people – like a crystal ball, you gaze in and get a glimpse of your future self. This is especially tough for people with young-onset Parkinson's, since you're right in the middle of life, advancing a career, raising a family – the idea of a fun retirement on a Costa Rican beach goes out the window and you start to wonder whether the life you're living is even worth it. A former governor in my state of Washington, Booth Gardener, was diagnosed with Parkinson's late in life, and he understood the struggle of people in the late stages of the disease. He advocated in the state legislature for the right of patients to die when these late stages took hold of their bodies. My hope is that I have at least 20-30 years before reaching that point in my life, and that there will be a cure for the illness by then. In addition, remember that not everyone progresses the same way – you are more likely to stay healthy if you make health and fitness a top priority. For someone diagnosed with young-onset Parkinson's today, the Costa Rican beach is still something worth hoping for.

Since being diagnosed, I know that I need to plan my life day-to-day rather than year-to-year as most people do. While others have the luxury of saying, "this is a project I'll take on next year" or "I'll think about going on that big trip in another year or two," I now must think more in the present and appreciate every moment. I need to keep telling myself "today I'll have more dopamine in my brain than ever again in the future, so live life now." Living this way has been both a blessing and a curse.

The Five Stages of Parkinson's

There are five stages to Parkinson's disease, and knowing where you're at can help you understand how your medication affects you, how exercise can benefit you, and how to tell if you're progressing to the next stage.

Stage I is typically when you get diagnosed with Parkinson's disease. You know that something's wrong, maybe a tremor or stiffness in your leg, you will go to the doctor and they will give you a diagnosis after a battery of tests. At this point, Parkinson's isn't affecting your life too much and you can still do most if not all of your daily activities. Usually at this stage, the disease is also invisible, so most people you interact with are not likely to notice that anything is even wrong. People who know you well and see you every day however may notice you dragging your foot, or that you don't smile or blink as often.

In Stage II, your symptoms start to get worse. If you had stiffness on the one side of your body, now it's affecting both sides of your body. This is when you notice both hands may have a tremor or that you are not able to type as well as you used to, or both feet are dragging a bit when you walk. Most people start having problems with posture – maybe you're slouching, bending yourself forward or backwards (Rosaline calls it the "backwards question-mark pose"). You are still able to work and do your regular activities, but you take more time doing them and they become harder to do.

In Stage III, you tend to have a lot more slowness in your movements and you begin to have loss of balance. You may begin to have falls or fall more often. You start to notice difficulty in getting dressed and buttoning your shirts or your pants. You may also have trouble eating because your fingers can't pick up that burrito or your hand shakes when you use a fork to pick up your pasta. This is also when you may start seeking help from other people to help you with your everyday activities. This is the time you may also start looking into using an assisted walking device to help avoid falls. You may also begin noticing that your medications are not working as effectively as they used to.

At Stage IV, the symptoms have become very severe and limiting for you. You may stop driving at this point, and you definitely find yourself needing help to do your daily tasks. At this point, you probably have stopped working and spend most of your time focused on your health and your disease. Emotional and cognitive decline is more noticeable, and your medications are likely not working at all, or if they are, your dosage is so high that the side effects have become unbearable. Perhaps you have changed your medication several times, and you're considering advanced therapies like DBS.

Stage V is the most advanced and debilitating stage in the disease. The stiffness and tremors may be so bad that you can't walk or even get out of bed. You definitely need help in doing everything from dressing to cooking to using the bathroom, and you will need a wheel chair for getting around. You have a lot of trouble swallowing and may even have a feeding tube installed. Cognitive and emotional symptoms have also worsened, and you're likely to be experiencing depression, hallucinations, even dementia.

It's important to again note that Parkinson's is a boutique disease, and that everyone experiences the disease differently and that it progresses differently in every case. This is just a general guideline and sometimes you may have varying symptoms at every stage. It's also possible to temporarily feel like you've progressed to the next stage when it's only a temporary flare up of symptoms due to stress. Progressing from one stage to another takes time, years in most cases, so don't become alarmed if you all of a sudden can't sleep or you have other sudden symptoms. If you pay attention to your body and track your symptoms over time, you will notice that you are having normal fluctuations that affect us all.

During my Stage I, I had severe balance problems that then disappeared in Phase II, and then returned more mildly later on. The same thing happened with my sense of smell. I have been fortunate to not have seious problems with my cognition, and I have been emotionally stable. In some ways, my body today at the middle of Stage II is doing better than when I was in Stage I, largely due to optimized medications, and a strong focus on exercise and diet.

Even at Stage V, it's possible to enjoy aspects of life. Having a human support system is extremely important at every stage, but during the final stages it can mean the difference between fading away, or going strong until the end. And at every stage it's also possible to enhance your health if you are not in good health. It's always possible to eat a little better, do a little bit of movement, and close your eyes to meditate. Fighting back against the disease is what we do. We are Parkinson's Warriors!

Causes

There is no consensus on what actually causes Parkinson's disease, and new research is coming out all the time. However, most agree that the likely cause is a combination of genetics and environmental effects. In other words, as I've heard it said by doctors, "genetics loads the gun, and the environment pulls the trigger." There are five gene mutations that are specifically known to cause a higher likelihood of Parkinson's, the LRRK2, PARK7, PINK1, PRKN, and SNCA genes. If you have used a genetic testing service like 23andMe, you can obtain your full genetic profile and search to see if you have mutations on these genes. Interestingly enough, only about 15% of PWPs have these mutations, so there are likely other genes that play a role and are yet to be discovered.

Three environmental factors have been linked to causing Parkinson's disease, though there may be more discovered after more research. The first environmental factor is concussions. Concussions occur when there is an impact to the head, causing the brain to swell. If you have enough concussions in your life and you have a genetic marker present in your DNA, you could develop Parkinson's, or a number of other scary neurological illnesses. It's generally thought that Mohammed Ali's Parkinson's was triggered by the blows his head received throughout his boxing career. Many retired professional football players have also developed Parkinson's and other conditions like Chronic Traumatic Encephalopathy (CTE).

Another environmental factor that has been identified as a potential cause of Parkinson's is heavy metal poisoning. Although this typically occurs in industrial settings like factories, the poisoning could happen in the home as well. These metals include lead – found in old water pipes and old paint, mercury, arsenic, and cadmium. Poisoning can occur due to air or water pollution, from canned foods, medicines, or through the ingestion of lead-based paints.

The third most common environmental factor shown to cause Parkinson's disease is pesticide poisoning. Many pesticides, like DDT, that have been outlawed for use in agriculture have been shown to cause cancers, infertility, Alzheimer's, and yes, Parkinson's disease. You may have been exposed to pesticides if you grew up on a farm, or if you were otherwise exposed to dangerous pesticides in agriculture or in home pest control.

I always wondered what caused my Parkinson's. Not that it matters now that I have it, but we always ask ourselves "why" and search for answers when these things happen. I don't appear to have the genetic mutation in my DNA, though I could have other DNA mutations that have yet to be linked to Parkinson's. There certainly is the possibility that an environmental factor played a role in my disease onset. As a kid, I had two mildly severe head injuries, neither of which caused a concussion. As a teenager and in my early 20s I worked in my family's business as a house painter, and I could have been exposed to poisonous industrial chemicals that triggered the illness. Lead paint was no longer used by the time I was working, but exposure could have happened when removing old paint from walls. Finally, there is the possibility of pesticide poisoning. In the late 1980s, my area of Los Angeles was sprayed by helicopter for a citywide Mediterranean fruit fly infestation. Helicopters flew overhead each night and literally sprayed pesticides over entire neighborhoods from above, and residents were instructed to stay indoors during the spraying times.

Any one of these factors could have, in theory, triggered my Parkinson's disease, or none at all. Recent research has added a new potential culprit by discovering evidence that Parkinson's begins in the gut. This means that it's possible that Parkinson's could be caused by something like bacteria or even an ulcer. This is a fascinating discovery if it turns out to be true. Regardless of what causes Parkinson's, you can't turn back time or cure yourself by undoing what is already done. Knowing the causes could help develop new treatments and could even lead to a cure, but it's best to look forward and think about how to improve your life with the disease, rather than dwell on what may have caused it for you.

Parkinson's Symptoms

There are many classic symptoms to Parkinson's disease. When James Parkinson's, the scientist the disease is named after, first recorded his observations about the disease, he noted three main characteristics that his patients exhibited; a tremor, shaking, or trembling, slowed movement, and stiffness or rigidity of the arms, legs, and trunk. There are a lot of other symptoms that PWPs experience, but we can start with these classic three.

Tremor is usually the first sign of Parkinson's in many patients. For many people, a tremor may start in the hands or feet and they may not think anything of it. Many people without Parkinson's can also have a tremor, for example when they start shaking during a fight-or-flight situation, or when their adrenaline is pumping after a car accident. What's not normal, is a resting tremor. A resting tremor happens when your hand is at rest, maybe on your lap or on a table, and your fingers start shaking or your hand begins moving uncontrollably. For many people, the hand tremor usually first manifests itself on a single finger or even fingertip. Many PWPs report a finger tremor as one of their first symptoms. A resting tremor alone, however, is not necessarily a sign of Parkinson's, as it's also a symptom of many other neurological conditions.

Slow movement is another symptom that is common in most PWPs. Slow movements usually begin on one side of the body and eventually affect both sides, and affect the fingers, arms, trunk, and head. Slowness of movement manifests itself on the face as a slow blink-rate, which may lead to dry or irritated eyes. Many people think at first that slow movement is due to aging, and while this may be true for the population as a whole as we age, the slowness is especially prominent in someone with Parkinson's.

Stiffness is another primary symptom of Parkinson's disease. Perhaps you have stiffness in your fingers, arms, legs, or feet. The stiffness feels like your limbs are just not wanting to move, and even an effort to specifically focus on that area and trying to relax your muscles will not work. Many doctors often view muscle stiffness as a symptom of something less severe. They may initially diagnose your muscle stiffness as a strain due to repetitive motion or other over-exertion. They may try to rule out any kind of injury by prescribing a pain medication or anti-inflammatory drug like Ibuprofen. If the issue resolves itself after this course of treatment, then the doctor will not investigate any further. But if this course of treatment doesn't work, then a responsible doctor will refer the patient to a neurologist for further examination.

As I was just 31 years old when I began seeing doctors for my left arm stiffness, they refused to believe that someone my age could have a condition like Parkinson's, so they tried different treatments during that time. At first, I was prescribed a six-month regiment of high-dose Ibuprofen. When that didn't work, they took x-rays and MRIs, sent me to an occupational therapist, and began suggesting herbal remedies. It wasn't until I demanded to see a specialist that the neurologist referred me to a movement disorder specialist, who eventually diagnosed me after his long examinations. My Parkinson's was difficult to diagnose, not only because of my age, but also because the stiff left arm was my only symptom for a very long time, while many with Parkinson's often exhibit more than one symptom early on.

There are of course many more symptoms of Parkinson's than just these classic three. PWPs all experience Parkinson's differently, and symptoms can range from constipation to cognitive decline, to loss of smell and even increased dandruff. I myself have experienced the well-known statue face where your face looks like it's frozen, usually in your sad face, which is not useful when you're trying to make new friends. I have also experienced toe curling as a symptom, which makes it difficult to put on shoes or walk when I'm completely off my medications.

Some symptoms are common to several neurological illnesses, so doctors often look for more than just a tremor before suggesting Parkinson's as a diagnosis. They can order blood tests, request MRIs or CAT scans, and put you on a trial dose of carbidopa-levodopa to test for response. In this phase, doctors are mainly trying to rule out worse diseases like Multiple Sclerosis, ALS, or Huntington's disease as much as they are trying to prove Parkinson's. Proper diagnosis is critical in order to receive the right treatment, but also to predict the disease's outcome in the long-term.

Prognosis

One of the first things you want to know once you are diagnosed with Parkinson's is, "Will I die of Parkinson's?" Let's just quickly answer that one: no, you will NOT die of Parkinson's. All things being equal, it's possible to live a life that is as long as it would be if you didn't have Parkinson's. You may then have a question like, "What kind of life can I expect in the next 5, 10, or 20 years?" The answer to this question, just like the answer to all of life's most important questions, is that it really depends.

Parkinson's is known as a progressive disease, which simply means that it gets worse over time. What this means is that, as time goes on, your symptoms will increase in number and severity. If you've just been diagnosed then you are likely at Stage I Parkinson's. At this stage, you may have a tremor, or slowness of movement, but within a couple years you may have stiffness in your legs, and increased tremor in your hands. The disease may also start only on one side, and then appear on the other side of your body as well. Everyone is different, and not everyone will have the same symptoms over the course of their disease.

Because the progression of Parkinson's disease is so difficult to predict, many people don't know how to plan for their futures. And while exercise is the only activity known to slow the disease progression, there is nothing that can stop it. This means that if you are currently working, you may not be able to work when the disease advances past a certain stage. Depending on your line of work, this may be at your time of diagnosis, or it can be in five or 10 years. The key is to keep your body as fit as possible in order to delay the progression and minimize the effects of symptoms.

Since there is no stopping the disease, many people decide to take the morbid move of planning for their demise. While this is a good life strategy in general, it's especially important for a PWP who has an uncertain future. The important thing here is to make sure there is a plan in place if anything should happen to you, but don't let it overtake your mind to make you feel like you are a terminal patient. You are not. It's always a good idea to have a will, decide on burial options and end-of-life directives, as well as have a sheet with all of your passwords, but then once that is done, you should forget all about it. That is for just-in-case. Your goal is not to live your life as a terminal patient, but to live your life as someone who has an illness but is going to do everything they can to fight it. There are two big killers with Parkinson's disease, and if you avoid them you can live a long life. Those two big killers are aspiration pneumonia and falls.

Aspiration Pneumonia is a breathing condition in which there is a swelling or infection of the lungs or larger airways. It happens when food, saliva, liquid, or vomit is breathed into the lungs or airways leading to the lungs, instead of being swallowed into the esophagus and stomach. Aspiration pneumonia can happen at any phase during the disease, but is most common in later stages when you begin having problems swallowing. This is why if you develop problems swallowing, your neurologist wants know about it right away.

Pneumonia can kill you if not treated properly and in time. Pneumonia can happen to anyone, and aspiration pneumonia can happen to anyone as well. However, it becomes more common in Parkinson's when you're swallowing function becomes impaired. The best advice to avoid this is to eat slowly, and eat foods that you know you can swallow properly. Some people in later stages consume liquid foods through a feeding tube to avoid this from happening. If you ever find yourself accidentally choking on a piece of food or choking when you drink something, and you develop problems breathing shortly thereafter, it may warrant a visit to the emergency room. Doctors can take x-rays to find if there is an infection.

Another common way of dying with Parkinson's is by taking a bad fall. It's no secret that we have problems with balance, and that this can affect walking. As we get older and bones become more frail, a fall that we could have absorbed in our early years can turn into something critical and even fatal. Falling during exercise or while walking up the stairs can lead to broken bones in your legs, hips, chest, or on your head. This could lead to other injuries like punctured organs. It's extremely important to protect yourself from falls by using an aide to get around if necessary. Don't hesitate to use a cane or walker to help prevent a nasty fall and to keep you from a visit to the emergency room. If fitness is an issue due to your balance, many local non-profits and hospitals offer chair yoga and similar fitness classes for those who are at risk for falls.

Physical Well-being

Physical fitness is important for anybody getting older, but it's especially important for PWPs. For us, being physically fit is the difference between falling and breaking an arm, and not falling at all or falling with minimal damage. I keep my body strong by taking part in a whole array of physical exercises during the week, all of which are discussed later on. Even if you're not big on exercise, you should at minimum be walking – even slowly walking just a few steps if that's all you can do – in order to keep the muscles and heart active. If walking is not a possibility for you, you should still find an activity that engages your muscles each day.

Although Parkinson's disease has no cure, there is one proven way to slow the disease's progression: physical exercise. I'll spare you the scientific background on this (though references can be found in the Appendix), but it's essentially a matter of "if you don't use it you lose it." We need to keep our muscles engaged and active, or we will become weaker and our disease will progress at a more rapid rate. The great thing is, even just a bit of exercise is useful in staving off progression. We don't need to become professional body builders or spend three hours a day in the gym. There is no reason to work out until you're exhausted. Just a few minutes of exercise each day can have a huge impact. Find a Parkinson's-specific exercise facility and work with a trainer to figure out how much exercise is ideal for you.

Emotional Well-being

PWPs tend to have problems maintaining emotional well-being, so it's especially important to pay special attention to anxiety, depression, and overall mood to maintain emotional stability. Mood is controlled by the dopamine in our brains, so it's no wonder PWPs tend to experience depression and anxiety at a higher rate than the general population. Dopamine is the chemical that makes us happy, and lacking dopamine leads to a down mood. This is why you are more likely to feel down in the morning before you have taken your medications. The good news is that, since depression and anxiety manifest themselves in PWPs due to a chemical deficiency, it's possible to regulate and even normalize mood with the right medications. Keeping track of your emotional health is just as important as tracking your physical health, that's why I keep track of my emotions and moods on a day-to-day basis. Treatments to regulate mood and fight depression and anxiety include talk therapy with a psychologist, medications provided by a psychiatrist, and meditation. It's also important to maintain a strong social network, as this has been shown to provide positive long-term effects.

Cognitive Well-being

Parkinson's affects cognition, as the brain mechanism that affects movement also affects our memory and problem-solving abilities. In addition to the disease itself, some medications like dopamine agonists can impair cognition. As with physical health, cognitive health is another case of "if you don't use it you lose it," so keeping the brain active with games, puzzles, and other cognitive exercises is very important. In later stages, some PWPs may inevitably experience a type of dementia specific to Parkinson's. Lewy Body Dementia can degrade the mind beyond what any medication or exercise may prevent, but by being proactive, you can slow its onset. Tracking your cognition over time through a series of recommended memory and logic tests can help you gauge your overall cognitive health.

In general, when it comes to the question of fitness, it's important to realize that everybody experiences the disease differently, and that each day with the disease is different. I have had periods where, perhaps for months, I felt like I was in serious decline. I felt like my disease was progressing much faster than normal. Often this has been during times of increased stress on my body and mind. During these times, I increased my physical fitness, meditated more often, and did everything I could to reduce my stress levels. I found that after a couple more months my symptoms had gone back to their former baseline, or only a bit worse. Just because you feel terrible one day or one week, it doesn't mean this will last. We have our ups and downs more frequently than people without an illness. Although there is not much we can do about that, knowing that it happens can help us anticipate and lessen the effects.

These ups and downs are the reasons why I'm such a proponent of tracking the illness on a day-to-day basis. By tracking the disease, we have an objective view of how our disease is progressing. This takes the emotion out of our tendency to self-diagnosis or over-react about a bad week, and it gives us a true bit of self-understanding. My wife, Rosaline, is a true believer in the objectivity of disease tracking. Whenever I'm having a bad week and I get overly dramatic and feel like the world is coming to an end, she asks me, "what does the chart tell you?" This is when I open up my app and look at my charts for physical, emotional, cognitive fitness, and notice that I'm likely not in a freefall decline, and that what I'm feeling at this moment is just a blip on my disease path.

Chapter III

Awakening Your Inner Parkinson's Warrior

"Know thy self, know thy enemy. A thousand battles, a thousand victories." – Sun Tzu

Sun Tzu was a strategist in ancient China, and his famous book, "The Art of War," is a classic book on winning in warfare. It's very strange for a pacifist like myself to be so adamant about waging war, but I sincerely believe that to fight Parkinson's, we must approach it with the mindset that we're going to war with an enemy. It's a war we didn't start, but it's a war in which we are fighting, whether we like it or not. There is currently no cure, so we're not talking about winning the war, but instead we're fighting to keep the illness at bay, and to not give up on ourselves and our way of life. To do this, we must awaken the warrior inside of us. We may not have ever shown the world the fury inside of us, but it's a fury that our Parkinson's will know, and that it will soon fear. This war is not easy for any of us, but it's one in which we must fight.

The Ballsy Palsy has met its match: it's you.

In order to make this fight truly fruitful, you must develop three aspects of your mind. First, you must have the motivation to succeed. Without motivation, the disease will take over and you won't even be able to begin the fight. Second, you must have the determination to succeed. There will be roadblocks and hurdles along the way – you should approach these roadblocks with a "bring it on" attitude. This is not a fight for the faint of heart, but we are already past that. Finally, you must show perseverance. There will be setbacks. There will be days you feel awful and won't want to get out of bed. You know this will happen, but you must never give up. It's possible to thrive while having Parkinson's disease, but to do so you must show up to fight the battles and be convinced of your resolve.

Going to War

Make no mistake, fighting Parkinson's is a long war. It will last a lifetime, it will have its ups and downs, and it may seem never-ending at times. But wars throughout history have lasted a long time, since both sides were determined to win and would not give in to failure. When we talk about going to war with Parkinson's, we really mean optimizing our lives so that the disease doesn't overcome us, but also that the disease doesn't rule our lives or define who we are. This is a delicate balance to achieve, but it can be done.

The war will be fought on many fronts. This second half of the book provides you the information and tools you'll need to succeed in your fight. In short order, I'll discuss building your army in the form of an experienced and caring team of people by your side throughout the journey. I'll discuss the ways you need to prepare yourself physically, emotionally, and cognitively. You will learn all about the weapons of this war; the medications, the exercises, the advanced treatments, the off-the-wall remedies, and the experimental therapies. I'll show you what has worked for many people, and what has not worked for anyone at all. At the end, you'll be armed with enough information to be dangerous, and you'll be prepared to build your own research library, you'll know how to search online for more answers, and you'll know how to ask better questions of your doctors.

Parkinson's doesn't have to take over your life; my life experience has hopefully proven this. My life is so much more than this disease.

As a thought exercise, I often ask people how they want to be remembered when they're gone. This may be a morbid line of enquiry, but I find it useful to those for whom I provide career and life counseling. There will be a line in your obituary that says "this person suffered from Parkinson's disease." As someone who has an as-of-yet-incurable illness, this line is unavoidable. However, the choice is yours during your life to decide if that will be the first line of your obituary, or if it will be the last line of your obituary. In other words, will your Parkinson's define you and your life, or will you be so focused on living a meaningful life that Parkinson's is relegated to the importance of a footnote in your overall life story? I want that sentence to be the last line of my obituary. I want my life to be defined by my love for my family and friends, for the contributions I have made to my community, and for the lives I have touched through my professional work. This is the reason I fight. I refuse to surrender to this ever-advancing enemy, and I refuse to be defined by it.

After Grief

When you are first diagnosed with Parkinson's, you will have a grieving period. The grief comes from the sense of loss – we feel like we've lost who we are, who we were, who we were meant to be in the future. We grieve for our loved ones, who will have also lost the lives they had, and who also face an uncertain future by being connected to a sick person. You will go through the five stages of grief – denial, anger, depression, bargaining, and acceptance, but then what? You will come out the other side of grief having accepted your diagnosis, but it doesn't mean you have accepted your fate.

This is why I believe there are two additional stages of grief when it relates to someone with Parkinson's – stage six: fighting back, and stage seven: advocacy. Together, these make up the "taking control" phase of the disease. We are well aware of the physical and emotional toll the Ballsy Palsy wants to inflict on us, and we have made the conscious decision to take control. First, we must learn to fight back – learn all about the disease, build an army of allies who will help you through the trenches, exercise to live a healthier life, develop a medication regimen, and fight the daily battles. After we have battled for some time and feel that we are much better off for it, we must now give back to our community in the form of advocacy – mentoring newly diagnosed PWPs, writing articles for local Parkinson's newsletters, taking part in medical trials, and generally, making your knowledge available to others in need. I'll discuss the ideas of fighting back and advocacy in the coming chapters.

Motivation

The first step to awakening your inner Parkinson's Warrior is to ignite your motivation. This may be easier said than done, since we PWPs are known for our apathy, another product of reduced dopamine levels. So let us begin by separating the keys to motivation into smaller pieces.

Set Small, Measurable Goals

Parkinson's is a big deal. Once you are diagnosed, it can become an overwhelming situation and take over your entire life. It's all you'll be able to think about for a while. Where do you start in taking care of yourself? How can you fight this illness and live a good life if you don't even know where to start? The first step is to make a small and measurable goal to get yourself started. The doctor said exercise is great for delaying disease progression. Ok, walk around the block every morning. They told you to eat healthier. Ok, cut out fried foods from your diet. Want to reduce stress in your life? Ok, stop for a moment each day at lunch to close your eyes and breathe deeply. These are small and measurable goals that you can make for yourself that, when combined, will lead to a healthier lifestyle that is beneficial for your overall health.

Develop a Mantra

What is the motto of your life? If you were an advertisement, what would be your slogan? Develop a mantra you can repeat to yourself and that gives you a sense of your best self. "I'll make it through this," "this will not defeat me," "I'm greater than this body tells me I am," are all great mantras to get you motivated. Whenever you're feeling down or feel that the disease is taking hold on a bad day, repeat your mantra to yourself. Say the words aloud and listen to them. Ingrain the thought into your head and believe it. After a while, you will embody this mantra; your body will know it subconsciously. You are strong, and you know it.

Commit Wholeheartedly and Publicly

It's easy to feel like giving in when you keep your thoughts to yourself and don't share with those who can keep you accountable. If you decide on an exercise routine or class, post about it online on your favorite social media site so that your friends and family know what you're doing.

By doing this, you're less likely to give up, mainly because you don't want to let down those who support you. Let your closest people know about your disease and tell them what you're doing to fight it. Not only will they be very supportive of you, they will also keep you accountable. They may even see you as an inspiration for reaching their own goals.

Maintain Your Optimism

Each day you will fight a different battle, and sometimes you will win while sometimes you will lose. It's important to not celebrate too heartily any big success, and not drown in self-pity when you have a failure. It's much better to keep your emotions level, and just tell yourself that this is how things will go today. Having a great day? Great, let people know about it. Having a really bad day? You know you will have these too, so don't be afraid to share these as well. Your people want to hear about your ups and downs; they want to support you. Believe it or not, when you give people the chance, they will stand up behind you to show their support. You need to remain positive and not let the bad things drag you down, nor let the good things send you over the moon. The more level you can practice keeping your emotions, the better you will handle the ups and downs as they come.

Determination

Determination is the firmness of purpose towards a specific goal. If your goal is to fight the war against Parkinson's, you must have a clear purpose and know what your goals are.

What Are Your Goals?

When fighting Parkinson's, your goals are likely to be to live a healthy, long life with minimum impact by the disease. Of course, you want to spend time with loved ones, travel, and live life to the fullest, but it all starts with maintaining your health and minimizing the disease's impact. Will it be difficult? Yes. Will everybody succeed at this? No. This is our ideal goal. Some of us will have it harder than others, but why not shoot for the stars? When I think about my goal with Parkinson's, I focus on the desire to remain healthy through exercise, diet, and social interaction until the cure is found or I die of old age. My goal is both broad, live long even with Parkinson's, and also specific, to exercise, eat well, and be social. This helps define my overall long-term strategy, as well as my short-term tactics to achieve that strategy.

Make the Decision

Once you have your goals set, it's important to make the decision to travel on the path that will lead to that goal. As PWPs, we sometimes find it difficult to make decisions, and often times our bodies try to make decisions for us. But it's important to tell our bodies that we are in control. Make the decision to live well with Parkinson's, and never look back. Keep yourself accountable. Put a sign next to your bed or computer, or make a wallpaper for your phone that says something like "I have decided to live well." This is different than your warrior mantra discussed earlier. This phrase is reminding you that you have made the decision to fight. Writing down your commitment phrase and keeping it where you can see it will serve as a constant reminder that you are a fighter.

Find Your Why

The simplest way to stay determined is to find your why. In other words, why are you doing this? Why are you fighting the battle against Parkinson's? Sure, you want to live a long and healthy life, but why? Perhaps you have a spouse that you want to spend as much time with, or you have grandchildren that you would like to see grow older. Perhaps you love to travel, and staying healthy means more travel in your life. Perhaps you have a bucket list that you need to complete before you're gone. Finding your why will keep you motivated and keep you determined to succeed. My why is that I love life. The experiences that I had before Parkinson's were amazing and I felt privileged to have had them. Living a healthy life means that I can have more memorable experiences with my wife, my friends, and my family. I love to travel and want to visit every continent and as many countries as possible. This is why I eat well, exercise as much as my body will allow, and would consider advanced therapies like DBS.

Prioritize Your Goals

Prioritizing your goals is essential and critical. If you say you want to be healthy and live a long life, yet you are working a stressful job long hours each day, you are not being true to your goals. We PWPs need certain things in our lives: low stress, healthy food, exercise, therapies, social interaction, etc. If you are not giving yourself what you need, you are not prioritizing yourself, which means you will never succeed in your goals. If your body asks for sleep, go take a nap. If you are at a party and you begin to feel tired, go home. If your body says no more alcohol or smoking, listen! The number one priority in your life is your health. If you're not fighting for good health, you're acting against your why.

Perseverance

Perseverance is all about continuing to move forward in the face of setbacks and disappointments. If something happens that makes you feel like the world is coming to an end, or maybe you're just having a bad day, persevering means that you have not raised the white flag of surrender. You will stop yourself before your emotions get out of control and you will allow yourself the time you need to recover. Once you have recovered and are at a place of peace in your mind, you will continue moving forward. Although this is listed as the last of the three skills you need in order to wake your inner Parkinson's Warrior, it's perhaps the most important. The reason is that, as a person with a chronic illness, you simply cannot give up. To give up with Parkinson's, is to give up on life. Therefore, you need to push through the bad times and reach the next battle. It's essential to move forward in the face of obstacles. It's much easier said than done, but it must be done.

Keep Your Why in Mind

One of the best and most effective ways to persevere is to keep your mind on why you are doing this. Remember your why. Whenever I see my wife come home from work, I remember my why. I want to be around her for as long as possible. I want to travel with her and have new adventures and make new memories. Whenever I think about that, my motivation and determination turn into perseverance and get me to go for a walk, avoid sugary drinks, relax and relieve my stress, and take my meds properly. Why did you decide to embark on this journey? Keep that reason in mind and you will find yourself moving forward.

Take Any Step Forward

When all hope seems lost and you have come to the point of almost giving up, taking any step forward can help break the curse. You were planning to go to the gym this morning, but then you began feeling bad and didn't go. Now you are in bed, feeling bad about yourself – the downward spiral has begun. Stop yourself now! Take any step forward by doing a couple of sit-ups or lift your arms above your head and hold them – all from bed. This is not the gym, but you are keeping the promise to yourself, you're moving. Maybe you are out to dinner with old friends, and you're enticed to eat fried foods and drink alcohol, even though you promised yourself you wouldn't. Take any step forward by drinking some water when you get home; this will help hydrate your body and also help digest the fried food. Taking any step forward, even in the presence of an apparent failure, is still a step forward. Doing this can help reset your mind to keep you moving forward toward your goals.

Go at Your Own Speed

Be careful of setting goals for yourself that you know you can't keep. Committing to going to the gym every day when you have never gone before is not realistic. Likewise, committing to cutting out all fried foods and refined sugars from one day to the next is setting yourself up for failure. Keep your goals in mind and take little steps. Life is a marathon, not a sprint. There is a long road ahead of you and incremental changes that keep you on track are better than big changes at which you will fail. Go at your own pace, and ignore the "common sense" advice from those around you, especially those without Parkinson's. Common sense advice doesn't often apply to PWPs. We're each different and you are your own special case in every circumstance.

I used to attend a yoga class with healthy young people, and I remember being disappointed at first, since I would not be able to perform the poses they were doing, nor could I do as many repetitions as the rest of the class. It was a bit embarrassing, to be totally honest. Then I thought to myself, "I'm here for me, not to look good in front of other people." So what if someone beside me could hold a plank pose for several minutes. I could hold my plank pose for 15 seconds, and that was good enough for me! I learned to ignore the instructions I knew were too advanced or strenuous for me, and from that day forward I did what I could and for as long as I could. I would not allow a stranger's judgement affect my exercise. Exercise is not a competition, but even if it was, it would only be a competition with myself. I have my own level that I call "Nick Level," which is different from Level 1, Level 2, etc. It's my level based on how I'm feeling that day, and it's different for each exercise.

Ignore the Negative Voices

You should ignore the negative voices that exist both inside and outside your mind. The little voice that tells you "I can't do this anymore," "this is too hard for me," "no one would fault me for giving up," – this internal voice is poison and should be ignored. It's easy to get down on yourself when you're facing a difficult and extremely challenging illness, but you need to keep those voices at bay. Think positive thoughts, consider your why, and take steps forward, even if those forward steps only move you a little bit. Of course, we will all have those days that we just want to give up and say "I'm done with today," and then go be in bed. That's fine – we need to allow ourselves those days as well. But you should never let those voices telling you to give up to take up any space in your brain for longer than just a little while. Substitute the negative voices with good thoughts about how you'll feel when you get to participate in your why.

The War is Never Ending

From this moment forward, you are a Parkinson's Warrior. You will fight epic battles each and every day, and you will win or lose with honor because you know the stakes. You will maximize your good times by filling them with your why, and in the bad times you will learn lessons and become a more formidable opponent. You will keep in mind that life is a marathon, not a sprint, and you have thousands of battles in front of you. There will be ups and there will be downs, and you will make it through as long as you fight. Remember, no one gets out of life alive. Your challenge is to live the best life possible and be the best you that you can be.

As with any war, the first step on the road to victory is to build an army. In Parkinson's speak, that is your care team.

Chapter IV

Your Care Team

Your care team is your first line of defense with everything related to Parkinson's. From seeking advice about medication interactions to having deep brain stimulation surgery, the people in your life and around you are the ones who will assist you with your care. You can't do it all alone. We need to allow others to help us, and we must be open to accepting help from others. Over time, you will develop a familiarity and trust with the professionals on your care team, similar to the trust you already have with your friends and family. While your care team undoubtedly has your very best interests in mind, keep in mind that every decision must ultimately be yours since it's your body and health. The advice from the professionals on your care team is invaluable, but be sure to be as informed as possible in order to have a debate and discussion for each step on the journey. Don't be ashamed to say "Let me do more research about this before I decide what to do," if you are not sure about a new treatment idea. Let's take a look at how these relations work, and learn how to get the most out of each of them.

Loved Ones

The people closest to you in your life, your friends and family, are at the top of the list as your first line of defense against Parkinson's. No one knows you and can support you like your friends and family. Keeping up with the most important relationships in your life is not only recommended, but required in order to live a long and happy life.

It's important to allow those who love you to help you throughout your journey. I'm not just talking about letting a loved one straighten up the house or cook dinner once in a while, but rather asking loved ones to accompany you to doctor visits. Things seem a lot less scary if you confront them with someone who cares about you. Each time I confirm an appointment with my neurologist or other specialist, I ask Rosaline to come with me, not only because she is smarter than me and can help ask better questions, but she also serves as a second set of ears and a second mouth to help the doctor get me the help I need. There are many times when she has jumped in when I couldn't remember the name of a certain medication or some other important detail. She also holds my hand and talks to me when I have blood drawn, helping me through the experience and keeping me from fainting.

I have found that it's best to be honest and open with loved ones about your disease. You don't have to let them know your day-to-day symptoms (unless they ask), and you don't need to tell them every time you are feeling down, but in general it's a good idea to make sure they know that you appreciate their support. If you are fortunate enough to have your spouse or partner as your primary caretaker, not enough can be said about the love and commitment they bring to your care. I have often publicly acknowledged that Rosaline is a saint for putting up with some of my ups and downs over the years. I draw strength from her own strength, as I realize that she goes through her own struggles living with a sick husband. Be sure your care partner gets the love and support they need as they accompany you on your journey.

Primary Doctor

Your primary doctor, also called a general practitioner, serves as your first stop on the way to specialists. Most health insurance policies require a visit to your primary doctor before allowing you to have a referral to a specialist. Depending on the severity of your illness, as well as where you live, your primary doctor may be very thorough in their examination and record-keeping, or they may just be a portal to other doctors. In the United States, my primary doctor took my vitals and conducted a limited neurological exam at each visit. In the Netherlands, my doctor still had not taken any vitals after nine months as her patient. My American doctor was more hands-on and involved in my overall treatment, while my Dutch doctor is more like a coordinator for my specialists. These are two approaches to primary care, and both have their advantages and disadvantages, mainly cost, quality, and overall approach to whole-health care.

Your primary doctor will likely be your first call if you are having any sort of non-Parkinson's related illness, or if you need to adjust any non-Parkinson's medications. In general, your primary doctor is not the person with whom you will be discussing your Parkinson's in depth, but rather they will have a general overview of everything in your medical history. It's worth repeating: your primary doctor will not be the person with whom you will be discussing your Parkinson's in depth. They should know about your Parkinson's by having access to your entire medical file, but your Parkinson's must be overseen by a neurologist, and preferably a movement disorder specialist. If you have Parkinson's, and your primary doctor says you don't need a neurologist or other specialist, run! I have known many people whose primary doctors refused to send them to a neurologist, especially in the early stages. Be sure you receive the referral you need, especially when you're dealing with HMO-style insurance systems. If you have asked for a referral and they have refused your request, ask for the denial in writing. This denial in writing is what you will need to file a complaint or to request a second opinion.

Movement Disorder Specialist

A movement disorder specialist is a neurologist who specializes in neurological diseases like Parkinson's and MS. If you can find a movement disorder specialist that is exclusively focused on Parkinson's, that's your best opportunity to receive the appropriate treatment. The movement disorder specialist will be an expert on Parkinson's, and will be able to track your disease, suggest medications, and give you general lifestyle advice. This person knows your disease better than any other professional, and after a while they will know you and your illness better than anyone else, so it's worth listening to their advice.

In general, a movement disorder appointment goes something like this: after checking in, the nurse takes your vitals and then you wait to see the doctor. The doctor will ask how you have been doing since your last visit, if you have any new concerns, and if there are any updates to your medications. They will perform a neurological exam on you. They will check your reflexes and sensitivity to touch, check the stiffness in your legs and arms, you'll touch your finger to their finger then to your nose and back again. They may want to see how you walk, and they might ask you to stand from a seated position without using your hands. This exam is called the Unified Parkinson's Disease Rating Scale, or

UPDRS. This is a standard exam that every movement disorder specialist uses to track your illness, and it's the same exam all around the world.

Your movement disorder specialist is your gateway to everything Parkinson's-related. They will suggest therapies and treatments, prescribe Parkinson's medications, and refer you to other specialists like counselors and physical therapists. In the early stages of the disease, you may see your movement disorder specialist once every 2 to 3 months, but after you have been put on a stable medication regimen, typically within a year from your initial diagnosis, you may see them once every six to twelve months.

Naturopath

A naturopathic doctor specializes in treatments that do not involve drugs or invasive procedures. Instead, they believe that the body can be treated using naturally-derived methods. While a naturopathic doctor is seen as an optional component of your care team – oftentimes health insurance plans don't include coverage for this type of treatment – I'd recommend having one to help balance out the traditional mainstream medical advice. This person will approach your Parkinson's disease from a holistic perspective. There are some naturopaths who know about neurology, but most will not and you will need to inform them about how Parkinson's has affected you. I was fortunate to have a naturopathic doctor in Seattle whose specialty was Parkinson's disease, and who had written books about treating Parkinson's holistically (more information in the Appendix).

A naturopath will ask you questions about your sleep, your diet, your exercise routine, and if you take any supplements. They may test you for things a traditional doctor may never consider, like vitamin deficiencies or for toxic levels of metals in your body. My naturopath tested me for heavy metal poisoning by taking a sample of my hair, and addressed my low energy level by giving me a shot of B12 vitamin. A second naturopath, who also happened to be a massage therapist, combined massage therapies with custom tinctures formulated to increase energy and improve mood. As you may have already noticed, a naturopathic doctor takes a much different approach than a traditional doctor. A good naturopath will be able to fill in the gaps of where traditional medicine leaves off.

It's important for your entire medical team to be aware of what each of them is doing, so be sure you share information among them to ensure avoiding dangerous interactions between medications and natural treatments. I was fortunate that my movement disorder specialist and naturopath actually knew each other, and they were aware of each other's approach to treatment. They often disagreed about the validity of a particular treatment, and it was up to me to make the decision of which to follow. Keep in mind that, no matter how experienced a doctor happens to be, no one knows all the answers, so it's best to do your own research and understand the benefits and risks of different treatments. This is especially true when working with a naturopath, whose treatments are often unsubstantiated by extensive clinical research, although that is changing as natural treatments increase in popularity.

Physical Therapist

A physical therapist is the person you will work with when a part of your body breaks down because of Parkinson's. For example, if you hurt your knee because you hit your leg against the ground too hard, the physical therapist will work with you to rehabilitate your knee, build muscle that will keep it protected from future injury, and perhaps also work with you on improving your walk. Over time, your physical therapist will get to know you and they will personalize your treatment to focus on your goals.

An extension of occasional and focused physical therapy is continuous general exercise with your physical therapist as personal trainer. Working with your physical therapist weekly to strengthen the body is a great preemptive measure to prevent complications like the dreaded falls. In these types of sessions, you work to strengthen your muscles so that if you do fall, you are less likely to seriously hurt yourself. In Seattle, PWPs were lucky to have one of the top physical therapists in the area open a Parkinson's-specific gym. The Parkinson's Fitness Project holds daily fitness classes in a gym with a beautiful lake view. If you don't live in Seattle, you can also subscribe to their fitness videos to do at home (link in the Appendix).

Occupational Therapist

An occupational therapist helps PWPs continue their day to day activities, including work and home activities, oftentimes supporting a recovery effort after losing the use of some part of the body. An occupational therapist specializing in Parkinson's will be especially skilled at working with hands, since tremors and stiffness often leave us with useless hands that can't type or have difficulty grasping objects. Occupational therapists could also help rehabilitate parts of your body that have atrophied due to lack of use. They can focus on gross movement by using mechanical grips, or work on fine movements with the use of therapy putty. These guided exercises are meant to improve strength and dexterity in your hands, two things that Parkinson's takes away.

Shortly after I had been diagnosed, but before I started taking carbidopa-levodopa, I had a lot of difficulty using my left hand and it became atrophied. I visited an occupational therapist who had me work with various types of putty meant to build strength in my fingers. This was very useful for keeping my hand active, but it was also very painful because the hand had been completely immobilized by Parkinson's, so moving it was a huge task that left me exhausted. Once I began taking medication for Parkinson's, the exercises became a lot easier, and so I switched to using the putty as a way to maintain my strength and dexterity in both hands.

Neuropsychologist

Neuropsychologists are concerned with the brain's relationship to behavior and cognition, and often work with PWPs to determine how both behavior and cognition change over time because of the disease. If you have Parkinson's, a neuropsychologist should be on your care team, since they understand the relationship between the disease and its non-motor symptoms like depression, anxiety, and mood. Most PWPs experience some form of cognitive or emotional issues during the course of their lives, so forming a relationship early on with a neuropsychologist can be extremely beneficial in the long run. Once you have established care, you can visit them on an as-needed basis, for those times when life really gets difficult, or continuously every couple of weeks to check in and keep on top of any issues as they develop.

Talk therapy is very useful for PWPs, especially when working with a neuropsychologist, since they can help you distinguish between something being circumstantial (i.e. depressed because you have Parkinson's) versus something that happens because of the disease itself (i.e. having feelings of depression because your medications are not working properly). Different doctors take different approaches, with some favoring just talk therapy during your sessions, while others will add in "homework," which means you have tasks to complete before the next session (ex. "List 10 things you're thankful for"). Different approaches work for different people and in different situations, so don't hesitate to tell the doctor if a particular approach is not working for you.

Neuropsychiatrist

While a neuropsychologist is more concerned with behavior and cognition as they relate to the brain and to Parkinson's, a neuropsychiatrist is more concerned with the intersection of Parkinson's and psychiatric disorders. A neuropsychiatrist will be less inclined to use talk therapy as a solution to depression, anxiety, and variations in mood, and they are more inclined to use psychiatric tools to determine if you are likely to need medication in order to treat these symptoms. It's clear that there is a difference between having occasional depression or down mood that can be helped with talk therapy, and having a chronic deep depression that has taken over your life and perhaps has made you have thoughts of suicide. A neuropsychiatrist can be especially helpful in the latter case, since they can offer you medications that have been proven to treat these more severe situations.

NOTE: If you currently feel you are severely depressed or have thoughts of suicide, please put down this book and call a suicide hotline or your local emergency number now! This is an emergency.

US: 800-273-8255   UK: 116 123   Other: Call your local emergency number.

Pharmacist

Your pharmacist is an important part of your team, since they can catch dangerous interactions between medications prescribed by different providers. For example, if you have a cardiologist for high blood pressure, and you also take Parkinson's drugs, along with an inhaler for asthma, the pharmacist will look at your prescriptions and let you know of any potential interactions. As a further example, there are some Parkinson's drugs that are dangerous to take with over-the-counter cough medication. This is why, even if I buy cough drops, I'll ask the pharmacist if there might be any interactions with my other medications. This simple step can easily save you a trip to the emergency room. Unfortunately for us PWPs, these situations can get us into trouble quite easily, so it's worth having a good relationship with the pharmacist, as well as trying to buy all of your medications from a single pharmacy that has all of your medical history and insurance information. Oftentimes, you may be taking so many medications that your pharmacist actually knows you by sight because they may see you there every week or two picking up something different. This is a good thing! The more they know you, the better they will be able to attend to your specific needs.

Support Staff

Support staff are any of the many people who work with your providers to coordinate care. For example, all of your doctors have receptionists working at the front desk, as well as nurses that perform the scheduling and coordinate medication refills. These are people you should be nice to and get to know, because you will be talking to them more often than you talk to your doctors. A good relationship with a doctor's assistant may mean the difference between getting an earlier appointment with a specialist because of a last-minute cancellation, or not. I know my neurologist's support staff by name, and I address them directly in my emails and ask to speak with them on my phone calls. Subsequently, whenever I need some kind of document for work or school, or I need a referral to do some kind of additional testing, they're very quick to respond.

Chapter V

Physical Fitness

My story of becoming a Parkinson's Warrior began with my decision to take my physical fitness seriously. It was the first step in my journey to better health, and for good reason. I cannot stress enough how important physical fitness is for PWPs. Physical fitness is the only thing known to help slow the disease's progression, and in general it will help prevent other illnesses as well. Don't forget that, just because we have Parkinson's, it doesn't mean we can't also be afflicted with another illness like heart disease, diabetes, or countless others.

Any exercise is worth doing, and I'd recommend you select an exercise that you will enjoy, and that you can continue doing (perhaps with modifications) throughout your life. Below are the exercises that are most commonly recommended for Parkinson's, all of which I've tried and can give you my own take on as well. Again, these are just recommendations. You should exercise at a pace and intensity that feels right for you. I recommend checking with your doctor before starting any exercise routine to be sure it's appropriate for you.

Yoga

If I could pick only one type of exercise for the rest of my life as someone with Parkinson's, I'd choose yoga. When some people think about yoga, they probably think about spirituality, the Indian origins of the practice, and perhaps think that yoga is something new-agey and weird. Although perhaps this may have been true years ago, today yoga is a common practice around the world and is perhaps the most effective physical exercise for treating Parkinson's.

The reason that yoga is so great for Parkinson's, is that the practice includes something for mind, body, and soul. The physical moves in yoga promote physical well-being. After a one-hour session of yoga, you will feel like you have worked your entire body, but not in an intense way like when using a treadmill or lifting weights. The best way I can describe yoga to someone who has never done it, is that it feels like getting a massage from the inside out. After a yoga session, my body feels relaxed and loose, and I notice improved movement and an overall feeling of well-being for the rest of the day.

Yoga also helps you find your emotional center by including meditation as a standard part of the practice. A good yoga instructor will make meditation an integral part of the workout, and they will guide you through meditations that will bring down your blood pressure, make you feel completely relaxed, and give you a feeling of oneness with the world. This doesn't have to have a spiritual element if you're not interested in that. Meditation gives you a feeling of general well-being and calmness in your mind. Your troubles seem to go away, and as you focus on your breath, you can feel your depression and anxiety lessen and your mood improve.

Although the physical and emotional benefits of yoga are more well-known that its cognitive benefits, yoga does indeed help sharpen the mind. A good instructor will work both sides of the body, switching from left to right, from hand to foot, and from up to down. Following along can be like a puzzle, and keeping up can certainly be a mental challenge. Some of the twists involved in advance yoga also seem like a form of puzzle, since you quite literally pretzel your arms and legs into different positions. Many of these advanced poses took me some time to understand, and I often relied on others showing me examples of how they were positioning their bodies before I could completely understand the poses. But the satisfaction of striking an advanced yoga pose and holding it for 5 or 10 seconds was extremely helpful for my mood and for my confidence as well.

The great thing about yoga is that anybody can do it. You don't need to be a completely healthy young person with rubber limbs to perform yoga. Each pose is individual to the person performing it, and even if you cannot stand or have poor balance, chair yoga can be an option as well. If you have advanced Parkinson's, there are still parts of yoga in which you may participate, such as meditation to help ease your mind. I highly recommend you attend a beginner yoga class if you have never tried it before.

My experience with yoga began right when I was diagnosed. My doctors told me that yoga could work miracles on my body, and so I enrolled in a yoga class at a local community college with a friend. It was not only fun to go to yoga twice a week, but it also gave me a chance to improve the bond with my friend, as he learned my limitations and better understood my disease. A class at a community college will be less expensive than a class at a yoga studio, so this is a great way to start your practice. These classes are usually very basic and open to anyone from the community. I'd recommend starting here, or at a community center where free classes are available. Once you have mastered the basics, you will want to find a yoga studio that offers an unlimited yoga membership where you can go every day if you want. This worked out well for me, since I stopped working full time and so had an open schedule to attend classes as often or as little as I wanted. The yoga studio I started out at in the Seattle area even had classes focused specifically on meditation, allowing me to further develop that aspect of my practice. After beginning a regular practice, I felt an improvement immediately and within a few months I felt better than when I was first diagnosed.

Tai-Chi

Tai-Chi is an ancient martial art of movement. It's often recommended by doctors and movement disorder specialists for its benefits to PWPs. The practice involves following an instructor slowly performing martial arts poses. Tai-Chi is all about slow, deliberate movement of the body from one position to the next. In essence, your body is flowing from one position to another. This helps PWPs by teaching how to control your body with intention rather than letting your body control you.

If yoga is too intense for you, Tai-Chi is a great alternative and I recommend it as a way to increase flexibility and strength while moving at a slower pace. While I appreciate Tai-Chi for its benefits for people with poor motor control, slow movements, and freezing, I prefer more high impact exercises and activities. However, this low impact may be just what you need if you suffer from arthritis and its related pains.

Cycling

There has been a lot of research done on cycling and its benefits for Parkinson's disease. Cycling for Parkinson's doesn't necessarily mean riding a bike outdoors. If you have poor balance, freezing, slowness of movement, or weak muscles, you could still benefit from cycling using stationary bikes (both single and tandem). This opens up cycling as an activity that most PWPs can do, and it's one of the activities that many in my local Parkinson's community enjoy. The act of cycling, pedaling using your feet and moving your legs in a circular motion, has been shown to improve brain function and decrease the severity of symptoms. One study showed that two people pedaling on a tandem bike, one person being a PWP and one without Parkinson's, benefited the PWP with improved movement and reduced symptoms for days after the cycling took place. The same benefits were shown using stationary bikes with motors that force pedaling at faster than average speeds.

More research needs to be done in this area, but one thing is for sure: cycling is extremely helpful for Parkinson's disease. My own experience with cycling has been mixed. During my teenage years, I was very much involved in cycling, and I was extremely good at controlling the bike. After being diagnosed with Parkinson's, I discovered that my poor balance had prevented me from safely riding a bike. The main issues are slowing down and stopping, since I'd be too slow in putting down my feet and maintaining the bike upright with one foot. This is when I decided to buy a stationary bike – nothing special, just a recumbent stationary bike that cost around $300 – and it worked wonders for me. I could feel an improvement in my symptoms as soon as I began cycling. Although I have since traded cycling for walking and jogging, I still highly recommend cycling to anyone with Parkinson's. If you can't ride a bike, a stationary bike will do. The important part is to push yourself beyond your average speed for at least several minutes. As always, check with your doctor if this is safe for you, and perhaps work with a trainer or therapist to ensure your safety.

Cycling is so good for Parkinson's, that many organizations have organized bike rides to help promote Parkinson's awareness. In my town of Seattle, there is a race called the STP: the Seattle to Portland race, in which riders bike for hundreds of miles on the side of the highway to raise awareness and money for charity. I'm amazed when I see PWPs participating in literally going the distance!

Walking

Walking can have similar benefits to cycling, and although one activity is not better or worse than another, they are different activities with different goals. Walking helps strengthen leg muscles, helps improve balance, and certainly provides a cardiovascular workout. Not only that, but it also helps clear your mind, especially if you can find a natural setting in which to walk. Walking is more appropriate for those who can't ride bikes, or for those who would like to slow things down for their fitness. Walking is generally low impact, and there can be a benefit even walking very slowly.

One of the reasons walking is so useful for balance is that walking helps train the small muscles in the bottom of the feet with each step taken. This benefit is increased by walking on uneven surfaces like an open field or on the beach rather than on a flat sidewalk. With every step, the small muscles on the bottom of your feet expand and contract, making them stronger. Once you take your shoes off at home, you will immediately notice a difference in your balance and in how you step. You will still have the poor balance from Parkinson's, but now your feet have strong muscles to help compensate for that poor balance.

My recommendation would be to buy a good quality pair of walking shoes. Preferably, go to a shop where they can test your gait, figure out how your foot is pronated, learn about your foot arch, and find shoes that will be a perfect fit for your feet. This will reduce the chances of tripping and falling, and will also make sure you have a smooth walk. If you have trouble walking or have extreme balance issues, I recommend walking with the assistance of a cane or walker.

Weights

While walking provides a great benefit for the lower body, exercising using free weights is a great way of strengthening the upper body. The upper body is the part we use most when we are rolling around in bed. Strengthening the arm muscles make it easier to turn in bed, and will certainly help with securing yourself to the grab bars in the shower or bathroom. The best way to start with free weights is with the lowest possible weight you can find – usually about two pounds. You can also use two full water bottles to stand in for weights. A 500ml water bottle weighs about 1.2 pounds, a great weight for absolute beginners.

There are four main dumbbell exercises I do in the morning. After warming up, I start with a set of 15 bicep curls, followed by 15 overhead presses, then 15 lateral raises, and finish with 15 upright rows. You can find YouTube videos to teach you the proper way to perform these exercises. These four exercises are enough to help maintain my muscle mass and keep me strong. Everybody is different, so you may do more or fewer repetitions, more or fewer exercise types, and more or less weight in your dumbbells. This is something a personal trainer or physical therapist can help you figure out.

Boxing

Boxing is a relatively new form of exercise for PWPs. It makes sense because boxing is an exercise that uses the entire body. Jabbing to either side moves the entire torso left and right, while the feet are also kept in constant motion. But it wasn't until a company called Rocksteady Boxing started doing these boxing classes specifically for PWPs, that the idea really took off.

Rocksteady Boxing runs fitness classes with boxing at its center. Here is my experience with the program: For your first class, you arrive early to register. You are then tested on several attributes: balance, memory, etc. They want to ensure you are healthy enough for the class and they are recording baseline measurements to compare with as your training progresses. You then get your own pair of boxing gloves, which are yours to keep. When the class begins, you start out on the floor like in yoga, waking up your muscles and getting warmed up. Then you take a place on a circuit with several stations where you can punch a boxing bag, run through different obstacles, and do things like pulling a really heavy rope. All these things keep you moving for about an hour and a half, and it's a lot of fun. It's also very intense, since you only have about 30 seconds to rest between each station. The coaches are all very encouraging and you work hard because you don't want to let them down.

I'll admit that this was the most intense type of workout I had ever done, even before Parkinson's. It's also difficult to modify workouts to suit your level, since you are moving quickly from station to station. With that said, I'd warn that Rock Steady is not for every PWP, but if you feel your body is healthy enough for a high-paced cardiovascular workout, then I'd recommend trying it to see if it appeals to you and your body. There are Rocksteady centers all around the United States, and many other countries have their own boxing-for-Parkinson's gyms as well.

CrossFit

What do you get when you cross weightlifting with cardio? You get CrossFit, something of a boot camp that throws in everything and the kitchen sink into your fitness routine. Typically, you are on a circuit with other people and with multiple stops along the way. At each stop, you perform some type of activity like throwing a medicine ball back and forth across the room for a minute or two, or pulling rope from one side of the room to the other. Then you switch activities by rotating your position with the whole class.

This is pretty intense exercise, and I'd not recommend that PWPs go to a regular CrossFit gym. In my city of Seattle, I was fortunate enough to have a specially tailored Parkinson's CrossFit class run by Parkinson's physical therapist, Nate Coomer, which was perfectly suited for PWPs of all levels. This special type of CrossFit includes cognitive drills that the regular CrossFit classes don't offer, and also includes Parkinson's-specific stretches that lead to improved flexibility, balance, and intentional movements. One of my favorite drills was moving my arms and legs while reciting a list of colors or letters. Another favorite was doing the exercises while trying to name every animal that starts with the letter A, for example, or counting down from 100 by 7s. This helped connect the cognitive with the physical, and was incredibly effective.

The reason this type of workout is useful for Parkinson's is that PWPs typically have difficulty coordinating between a thought and a different action, like chewing gum and walking at the same time. I notice my physical symptoms worsen whenever I need to think about something else at the same time I try to move. This is a skill we need to focus on maintaining and even improving over time, but which gets little attention in traditional exercises. No matter what type of exercise you do, there should be a cognitive component to it as well.

Dancing

An interesting fact about Parkinson's is that the act of freezing, which happens with at least half of all PWPs, can be disrupted. For example, you can buy a walker fitted with a laser that creates a guide path directly in front of it, giving the PWP a visual indicator of where their foot should step next. The laser guide disrupts the pathways in the brain that want to freeze your gait, and it allows you to step without freezing. Music is known to have a similar effect on the brain as the laser guide, but it works through the auditory system rather than through vision. In fact, a musical beat works so well to disrupt freezing that some PWPs carry metronomes or listen to music to improve their gait. This is why dancing is so popular in the Parkinson's community.

Dancing to a rhythm is not only good exercise, but it has a social component to it as well. Many nonprofits put on weekly or monthly dances for PWPs and their partners, and these are extremely popular. But you don't need to go to one of these dances to reap the benefits. Put on an album at home, get up, and move! If you're paying attention to the music, your body gets tricked into moving on the beat and you can move without freezing. It's quite amazing, actually. I'm not saying that music will turn you into a great dancer or that you will even be at all graceful in your moves, but you will notice that the freezing is minimized or disappears completely.

Singing

While we know that Parkinson's is a movement disorder, one of the movements that are limited with the illness, but which is not discussed often enough, is vocal cord control. The vocal cords are just as affected by weakness, stiffness, and even a shake, as your hands and feet. Over time, PWPs become quieter to the point where it can be difficult to hear them speak, especially in loud places. Taking the right medication and being "on" helps to improve your voice, but you can also exercise your voice regularly by using it to sing.

Singing is probably one of the best vocal exercises because it's easy to do. Whether you are in the shower or in the car, you can sing along to the radio. The goal is to be louder than you normally think you should be. You try to reach a volume in your voice where it feels like you're almost yelling. Doing this for half an hour to an hour each day can help improve loudness in your voice as the disease worsens.

Another method to exercise and strengthen your voice is called Loud (a part of the LSVT Big & Loud therapy program), and it aims to improve voice quality in PWPs with a set of routine exercises. Therapists train you during sessions to use a loud voice at all times. You perform practice drills for loosening your vocal cords, and the therapist makes you repeat written passages using a very loud voice. The PWP usually attends sessions twice a week for six or eight weeks, and the program can be repeated every year or two as the disease progresses.

An interesting take on singing as a therapy for Parkinson's is the barbershop quartet of PWPs in Seattle called the Tremolos. They get together and practice their loud voices singing songs, and sometimes they even perform for others. Not only does this provide a therapeutic experience for the singers' voices, it's also a social activity that gets PWPs out of the house and doing something fun and engaging. Search YouTube for "Parkinson's Tremolos" for some fun and heart-warming videos.

Something Unconventional: Pinball

One unconventional type of exercise in which I personally participate and recommend to others is pinball. Yes, I'm talking about the wooden machines with the flippers and the silver ball. Not only is playing pinball a fun and challenging pastime, when done right, the player uses their entire body to keep the ball in play. Different machines have different rule sets, so once you have mastered one, there are hundreds more to master, making this a cognitive exercise that helps sharpen your mind while also working on your hand-eye coordination and reflexes. Although my short-term memory is often pretty terrible, I'm able to remember the rules to different games, and I notice my short-term memory actually improve on the days following some intense pinballing. Pinball can be such a physical activity that after some intense pinball tournaments, I left sweating and felt tired the next day. I highly recommend finding an arcade in your neighborhood or even just a bar with a single machine and try playing it.

Do What Works for You

Ultimately, physical fitness is a personal activity. You should do whatever comes naturally to you, and whatever makes you feel good. Remember, everybody is affected by the disease differently, so you may not be able or willing to participate in walking or dancing or cycling. That's okay. I have a friend who plays pool several times a week. Perhaps that activity doesn't get your heart racing like aerobic exercise, but he still stretches his body as he lines up the shots, and he must also exercise his cognition when deciding what shots to take. It works for him. Another friend plays golf weekly – it's another low impact exercise, but it involves walking from hole to hole, and using the whole body to swing at the ball. He may not get the best scores, but he is out there moving his body and having a good time. I also have several friends who enjoy swimming. They're not using the diving board, and certainly don't swim in the deep end, but they are moving their bodies freely in the water, and the water's resistance makes for a great workout.

My advice is to do whatever works for you. If you hate lifting weights and can't stand jogging or walking with no destination in mind, you are less likely to continue doing it in the long term. Instead, if you pick an activity that you enjoy and that brings happiness to your life, you're more likely to stick with it. Your doctors will certainly ask you what kind of fitness you do each week. I get a kick out of telling them that I play pinball and arcade games, then explain to them the benefits and seeing them realize that these really are physical activities. This also broadens their minds, which may lead to them suggesting these activities to other PWPs as well. In fact, one person told me that their neurologist had suggested for her to play pinball because another patient of hers does it. The PWP responded, "oh, that's Nick Pernisco!" That brought a smile to my face.

Tracking Physical Fitness

As with everything related to Parkinson's, it's important to track your fitness on a regular basis to note any changes, positive or negative. You can use my Parkinson's LifeKit app, a spreadsheet, or even just a small journal. The

Parkinson's LifeKit app allows you to test your daily physical condition through a central nervous system test. The test asks you to tap a button as quickly as you can for ten seconds. This tap test can reveal a lot of information about how your body is doing at that moment. Alternatively, you can keep track of any kind of marker that works for you. How many steps you walk per day for example, or how you feel, on a scale of 1 to 10, before and after doing a few sets of weights with dumbbells. Track this information over time so that you get an idea of where your health is headed. For example, if you notice that over the span of six months your number of steps per day has trended downwards, you will have objective data that you could bring to your neurologist to discuss. This analysis may help determine if you need to make changes to your medication or make some other change to your routine.

Chapter VI

Emotional Fitness

Just like physical fitness, emotional fitness is extremely important for PWPs. Depression, anxiety, and stress can wreak havoc on your nervous system and on your mood. Recognizing this is the first important part, then you can figure out what to do about it.

Depression

Depression is actually a very common emotional symptom for PWPs. In fact, looking back to my first days of feeling out of the ordinary, it was clear that my first symptom of Parkinson's was depression. The reason this occurs is because the chemical your brain uses when feeling joy is dopamine, the same chemical that is depleted with Parkinson's. This means that depression in Parkinson's, especially pre-diagnosis, is likely not psychological, but rather chemical. As your brain has less dopamine to work with, you are less likely to experience happiness or joy, and it may take a lot more to have those feelings.

Depression in Parkinson's can be treated in two main ways: talk therapy with a psychologist is useful for helping to come to terms with having Parkinson's and adjusting to "the new normal" of living with a chronic illness. The second way of treating depression in Parkinson's is with antidepressant medications. Since PWPs are deficient in the chemical meant to help feel happiness, introducing a chemical to help balance out the brain makes sense. I'm not a fan of taking unnecessary medications, and if I thought that this could be helped completely with talk therapy or by changing my perspective on life, or by taking my afternoons off to stroll in the park, I'd prefer that. Unfortunately, Parkinson's and its effects on the brain don't work that way. Speak to your neurologist to find out if antidepressants are right in your situation, or reach out to your neuropsychiatrist to discuss more targeted therapies.

Anxiety

Anxiety has many causes, but with Parkinson's it can be a side effect of the disease, or it may also be caused in part by our feelings about the disease. For example, a typical type of anxiety in PWPs is being in public and other people noticing that they have an illness. For example, when you go to a restaurant and you have trouble eating with your hands, this may cause anxiety because you may feel that people are watching you, or you may not feel comfortable eating in public in general. This is one of the reasons I don't eat burritos or hamburgers in public anymore! You may also feel self-conscious because you have difficulty walking or you aren't able to smile or nod during a conversation. Feeling like you're constantly being watched, and judged, by other people is no fun.

Another type of anxiety may be more related to general worry about the direction of your disease progression. You wake up in the middle of the night and start thinking – where is the disease going, how will you feel tomorrow, or the next day, or in a year? Suddenly, the hamster in your brain is on its wheel and you can no longer sleep. This type of worry leads to severe anxiety that can really affect your quality of life. Typically, your neurologist or a neuropsychiatrist can prescribe antianxiety medications. One well known and well tolerated anxiety and depression medication for PWPs is Venlafaxine, which is discussed in the medications chapter.

Stress

Stress and anxiety are closely related, but stress typically comes from your current situation, and could be reduced by making lifestyle changes. For example, you may feel more stress at work because you feel you're underperforming, or you're being seen by others as underperforming. You might have stress at home because of conflicts or tension with family members or friends, or because you're not making ends meet due to lack of work. Stress unfortunately worsens Parkinson's disease symptoms, and could cause the disease to advance more quickly. It's key in Parkinson's to reduce stress as much as possible. Reducing stress can lead to great reduction of symptoms and can lead to a better quality of life.

Reducing stress with Parkinson's can be a bit of a chicken-and-egg situation. You may be stressed because things in life are getting difficult for you, but things in life are difficult for you because you're stressed. If you learn to reduce stress, perhaps through yoga or another physical activity, or through medication that reduces anxiety or depression, your life could drastically improve, which will lead to reducing the amount of stress you feel. It's worth making the effort to reduce stress, as it will lead to a longer, healthier, and better life.

Mindfulness

Mindfulness is all about living in the now rather than in the past or in the future, and about savoring the moment.

We tend to live our lives thinking about the past, and perhaps how good it used to be before we were diagnosed, or thinking about the future and how our bodies will decline over time thanks to the disease. Many of us who say we live in the present are really just involving ourselves in endless and unimportant tasks meant to keep us busy, but we still miss the big picture. It's important to stop every once in a while, "smell the roses," as they say, and look at the big picture. Look at the world around you, how beautiful nature's colors are in different seasons, the new clothing your partner or your family or friends are wearing, the smell of fresh coffee or tea, the sounds of people having a conversation, the warmth of the morning sun on your skin, the taste of your favorite food – what are those ingredients you're tasting?

Mindfulness is all about experiencing life in all of its glory and with all of your senses, all while staying in the present. This can have a powerful effect on our bodies and our minds. By focusing on our sensory experiences, we are not focused on the things that preoccupy us. People who practice mindfulness, whether they have Parkinson's or not, often seek to experience all that life has to offer. For example, travel is seen as a highly desirable experience in many people's lives. There's something to be said about having new experiences in new places, with new people, and learning new languages, and seeing how these experiences can have a positive effect on our lives. Having new experiences, and then focusing our thoughts on those experiences, can actually have a physical effect on our brains. Learning new things has long been known to increase plasticity in the brain. So even at an older age and with advanced Parkinson's disease, you can create new connections in your synapses and improve your brain. This is all part of mindfulness.

Meditation

The one activity I have found to be most helpful, likely because it can be done at any time, is meditation, with the intention of releasing negative emotions. I could meditate when my meds are "on" and I'm having wild dyskinesia, or when I'm completely "off" with tremors and stiffness. In either case, I can close my eyes and meditate. Many associate meditation with spiritual experiences, but it doesn't have to be. Meditation is the technique of freeing your mind of all thoughts and just being. This helps calm the mind and body and helps to reduce symptoms and side effects to a certain degree.

I remember having a severe case of pneumonia around Christmas of 2014. I was having a very difficult time breathing and my body felt sore beyond what the usual Parkinson's would offer me. I was in extremely bad shape and would end up going to the emergency room. But before it was time to go to the hospital, I was lying in bed, full of pain and unable to breathe properly, and so I closed my eyes and tried to clear my mind. I forced myself to take long, even breaths, and focused my thoughts on the sound of that breath. Within 30 seconds, the pain felt like it had left my body and I felt a subtle comfort deep within me. My breathing had been so horrible that I could actually feel it coming under my control. The meditation helped quell my pneumonia symptoms until Rosaline could get home and take me to the hospital. This is just one example of how meditation can help calm your body and mind. There is certainly a mind-body connection, and meditation proves it!

Here's how I meditate: wherever I am, I try to sit or lay down if I can. Then I close my eyes and focus on the sound of my breath. I shut out every sound and every movement outside my body and my surroundings – I simply focus on the sound of my breathing. It often helps me to put a hand over my sternum so I can also feel the up and down movements of my chest as my breath goes in and out. I focus on my breathing, then purposely try to slow my breathing to a breath (full inhale and exhale) every 5 to 7 seconds. Since I'm focusing on my breath, I'm ignoring everything else that's around me. Suddenly my body becomes calm, and I feel like I'm just floating in space. After a quick meditation session of 5 to 10 minutes, I have the sensation of being refreshed and I feel clarity and calmness in my mind. If I meditate for 30 to 60 minutes, I may be able to regain some energy to do more activities that day.

Support Groups

Support groups can be great for people who have just been diagnosed, and for those who feel like they need to connect with others who have their same illness. Parkinson's support groups are very useful because the disease is so rare relative to other diseases, that you are unlikely to find someone with Parkinson's in your everyday life. Connecting with others and sharing experiences and tips on medication and exercise can have a positive effect on your life. It's also a good way to meet people at different stages of the disease and learn about how they live their lives. This is especially useful if you feel anxiety or worry about going out in public with people who may not understand you or may not understand your disease. Your Parkinson's support group is a great way to escape all of that and spend time with people just like you, struggling day-to-day but wanting to live full lives as much as possible. I have met a lot of great people in the support groups I've attended. Some of my friends are people I would not have otherwise met if not for the fact that we were in the same situation. I've made friends with teachers, farmers, lawyers, businesspeople, and from every walk of life imaginable, and it's the illness that brought us together. I've met people who are very much into cycling, and others who enjoy having drinks at the bar. Through my support groups, I have developed an entire social network of people who come from different parts of life and have come together to share ideas and thoughts on Parkinson's.

With that said, support groups may not be for everyone. It can be challenging for us to see others who are more advanced in their disease. It's easy to convince ourselves of the worst-case scenario, meeting someone in really bad shape and thinking "this could be me in five or ten years." This could actually make things worse and lead you down the path of depression. Of course, everyone progresses at a different rate and not everyone experiences the different phases of the disease in the same way. But this can still be very difficult for some people to experience. Another difficult aspect of support groups is that I have been going to them long enough to have met people who have passed away in the course of me knowing them. Before support groups, I had not known anyone who had passed away, mainly because of my younger age and good fortune. You might hear the news from the support group leader and think "she was only 15 years older than me and she seemed alright the last time I saw her." That can be a tough situation to accept. At the same time, I have met some very strong and amazing people, and I do not at all regret meeting those wonderful people who I only had a chance to know for just a while.

Overall, the support group experience has been a positive one, and if you are deciding if a support group is for you or not, I'd recommend trying it. It has been my experience that Parkinson's support groups are very welcoming and provide insights that are not available anywhere else, even in online support groups. If you are looking for a support group to join, I'd recommend checking with your local Parkinson's non-profits to see what kind of support groups they offer. Check the resources section at the end of this book for some links. If you live in a rural area or in a smaller city, you may also want to look into joining an online support group, such as those that are on Facebook or are part of an Internet forum on a non-profit's website. While I prefer to meet in real-life support groups, online groups are a great way to get to know more people from around the world and get even more perspectives.

Tracking Emotional Fitness

As we have seen, it's clear that PWPs experience emotional swings that can change day to day or week to week. Part of our emotional swings have to do with the fact that we have an incurable illness, and part of it is also a chemical imbalance due to changes in our dopamine receptors. When we are unmedicated, it's easy for those feelings of depression or anxiety to seep in, while when our meds are on and working we tend to feel more upbeat and positive. We know that this is normal in the disease, and although we want to try to be as upbeat as possible as often as we can, having mood shifts is not typically something to be worried about on a day-to-day basis if properly treated. However, tracking our emotional state on a day-to-day basis can reveal long-term patterns that can give us an early warning of severe depression or other emotional problems that could lead down worse roads.

Oftentimes, neurologists will conduct an emotion or mood survey during your appointment in order to gauge where you are emotionally at a particular point in time. They will ask questions like if you have had thoughts of suicide, or feelings of hopelessness. The problem with these tests is that they are being asked about your recent mood, for example in the last week or two. It would be more useful to have a more granular look at your mood by recording it every day. This way, not only can you see how you are doing in the last day or two and see the ups and downs more finely, but you can also detect overall trends over one month or even over six months or longer.

My Parkinson's LifeKit app has a built-in emotional fitness tracker. It's a modified version of the survey given by neurologists and therapists, and it's adapted to be used as a daily check on your emotional state. It includes questions about your general mood, about your appetite, and about your sleep. After answering these questions, the test will record your score, which then can be viewed in the greater context of longer periods of time. If for example, you get low scores consistently over the course of a month, it may be a warning sign that might call for a visit with your medical team.

My own experience tracking my emotional state shows some very interesting results that have contributed to my understanding of how Parkinson's affects me. For example, I know that there are days that I wake up and just want to stay in bed, not because there is anything physically wrong, but maybe because it's just gloomy outside. If it happens two days in a row, it's easy to overreact and say maybe this is some new depression of some sort. However, I can bring up my chart for emotional fitness and see that this recent low mood is just a little dip in an otherwise positive emotional state over time. The next day when I feel a lot better, I record that score as well, and my average emotional score moves up, indicating that yes, the past two days were just a little blip, and likely insignificant in the long run. This can only be accomplished by keeping track of these emotional markers on a daily basis.

Chapter VII

Cognitive Fitness

Cognitive deficiencies are part of what are considered non-motor symptoms in Parkinson's. The disease itself, as well as the use of certain medications, can cause cognitive difficulties like a decline in short-term and long-term memory, an increase in compulsive tendencies, hallucinations, vivid nightmares, as well as dementia. It's important to track these changes over time and note when they increase or decrease.

Memory

One of the most common declines in cognitive fitness with Parkinson's is with short-term and long-term memory. This usually happens due to the disease itself, but can also be exacerbated by certain medications like dopamine agonists. Carbidopa-levodopa can actually improve short-term memory. This improvement can be experienced by taking a memory test while unmedicated in the morning, and then repeating the test later in the afternoon when you feel your medications are at their peak. You will notice an improvement in memory and you'll find that you are retaining more information. Learning new things can be difficult for PWPs, so it can be useful to coordinate learning with when your medications are at their most effective.

Thinking

Thinking can also be affected by Parkinson's. The ability to think, concentrate, focus, and organize your thoughts are all affected by the disease itself, and also by medications like dopamine agonists. Just as with memory however, carbidopa-levodopa can help improve thinking as well. It's also useful to keep your mind active, perhaps doing puzzles or by watching television game shows. Anything you can do to keep your mind active, especially as you age with the disease, is useful in preventing or delaying the decline in thinking and concentration.

Decision Making

A classic cognitive symptom in Parkinson's is a decline in decision-making ability. Some minor symptoms include difficulty in choosing a type of cereal at the market or choosing whether to go out or stay in on a particular day. However, these small annoyances of indecision are nothing compared to an impairment that causes the inability to make split-second decisions, like while driving a vehicle. Combining the inability to make split-seconds decisions with slow movements and reflexes is a recipe for disaster. This is why many PWPs choose to stop driving after a certain point in their disease. The decline in decision-making ability usually comes from the disease itself and not from medications, but some medications may worsen the decline. Combining physical fitness with cognitive exercises, as is often done in Parkinson's-specific exercise classes, can help delay the decline of this symptom.

Compulsion

Dopamine agonists are known to cause compulsive behaviors in people, and can lead to dangerous situations. I have heard stories of people gambling excessively and losing their entire life savings, people's sex compulsions leading them to have sex with prostitutes to satisfy those urges, and doing other activities that have gotten them into dangerous situations. Your neurologist may offer you the assurance that dopamine agonists are well tolerated, and in general that may be true, but if you are a part of that percentage of people who have these compulsive side effects, life can get quite unpleasant. I'm not suggesting that you shouldn't try dopamine agonists, but be aware of the side effects. If you do decide to take dopamine agonists, it's certainly useful and prudent to keep track of any compulsions you experience.

Hallucinations

Some medications are known to cause hallucinations, while hallucinations may also be potential signs of the beginnings of Lewy body Dementia. Typically, hallucinations include hearing or seeing things that are not there, and not realizing that these are hallucinations. You may hear noises or a voice when you are alone, or you may see a figure or movements when no one else does. Neuropsychiatrists differentiate between hallucinations you experience and know are not real and hallucinations you experience and accepting them as real. A couple of years ago I was hearing my mother's voice when I'd go to sleep. I knew she was not actually there, and I wrote the hallucinations off as anxiety or stress-induced. After about a month, the hallucinations went away and never came back. My neuropsychiatrist told me this was likely not something to worry about. If you begin experiencing hallucinations and believe they are real (as recognized and confirmed by your care partner), immediately contact your neurologist or neuropsychiatrist and let them know. This can be a very serious development.

Vivid Nightmares

Sleep disturbances are a part of Parkinson's, and vivid nightmares are a part of that aspect of the disease. Many PWPs have trouble sleeping at night, rollover often, wake up in the middle of the night for various reasons, and most importantly, have vivid nightmares and sometimes act out those nightmares. For example, I have had nightmares in which I'm in a fight, and I'll kick in my nightmare and kick my leg in real life as well. Knowing this, I now try to sleep on my back or on my side against the wall so that I don't accidentally kick Rosaline in the middle of the night. Many PWPs take melatonin to help sleep at night, though you should check with your doctor before starting melatonin since it can have interactions with other medications.

Dementia

Dementia occurs in a certain percentage of PWPs. Dementia includes many of the cognitive issues mentioned above, along with confusion, forgetfulness, and other severe cognitive symptoms. Only a neurologist can diagnose dementia, but diagnosis can be clearer and more definitive if you track various symptoms over time. For example, if hallucinations and forgetfulness have increased in the past year, this may be an important development that your neurologist should know about.

Practice Active Cognition

It's very important to keep your mind active as you age, especially as you age with Parkinson's. Allow yourself the time to practice mindfulness, and also exercise your cognitive functions. Watch your favorite game shows on television, do crossword puzzles, learn a new language, expose yourself to new things like art, keep a notebook with your thoughts, or learn something new like math or astronomy. All of these things will help improve your cognition, and could help delay the onset of more serious symptoms.

Tracking Cognitive Fitness

Tracking your cognitive fitness is essential with Parkinson's. Often, we could be having a bad day in which our minds are not working as we expect, and it would be useful to know whether this is just a short-term situation due to stress or a new medication, or if this is a new longer-term development we should be worried about. You can track memory and logical problem-solving capabilities with the Parkinson's LifeKit app. Parkinson's LifeKit allows you to track your memory with a memory game you can play on a daily basis. The task is to turn over and match pairs in a deck of 16 cards. The faster you can solve the puzzle, the better your memory is at that moment. You can also track your problem-solving abilities with the daily Stroop-style test. This test shows you an ever-changing reference color, and you are tasked with tapping on that same color on the grid below. After a while, the test becomes more complex by trying to trick you into selecting the wrong color. Doing this will give you two objective data points to follow your cognitive abilities on a day-to-day basis and over time.

Chapter VIII

Nutrition

Proper nutrition is such an important part of a healthy lifestyle, especially as we age, but it's especially important for those of us with Parkinson's. The food we put into our bodies could ease symptoms, or it can make symptoms worse. Proper diet could also help combat inflammation and might actually help slow the disease's progression, while other foods could leave us in worse health and make the disease progress much faster. Nutrition is more than just getting your vitamins and minerals in your meals. Good nutrition involves eating the right foods at the right times of day, and for reasons beyond simply filling our stomachs.

Neuroprotective Foods

The best place to start with nutrition is in discussing foods that have neuroprotective properties. Eating foods packed with nutrients and antioxidants will not only contribute to your overall health, but will also help protect against the progression of Parkinson's. This is done by combatting free radicals, the things responsible for premature cell degeneration and death, with antioxidant foods. Foods filled with antioxidants include green vegetables like spinach and broccoli and fatty non-meats like avocado, olive oil, and nuts. You want to minimize animal proteins, since these produce free radicals. This type of diet also includes eating grains and legumes, drinking lots of water, and avoiding processed foods like sugar and deep-fried starches. This diet is healthy, neuroprotective, and will taste delicious when done right.

As a comparison, diets high in red meat, processed foods, and sugary drinks lead to diseases like heart disease, diabetes, and more. Red meat in particular causes inflammation and the release of free radicals in the body, which leads to brain cell degeneration. Remember, as someone with a chronic illness, you want your body to be as healthy as possible, and it all begins with what you put into your mouth. Let's take a look at these food categories individually.

Caffeine – Coffee and Tea

There are some studies that show that caffeine can have a neuroprotective effect. Not only has the consumption of coffee and tea been shown to delay the onset of Parkinson's, it has also shown benefit in people already diagnosed with Parkinson's. Caffeine is a drug and can give you a buzz or a high, and there is definitely some interaction between caffeine and the dopamine receptors in our brains. Caffeine can help jumpstart our brains and ease the absorption of medication like carbidopa-levodopa and dopamine agonists.

I have personally had mixed results with caffeine. I do feel like my brain works better when I consume caffeine, and I especially notice improved cognition. However, caffeine amplifies the effects of carbidopa-levodopa, leading to more numerous and intense dyskinesias than normal. Often when I need to use my brain for some especially intense cognitive task like writing, teaching, or programming, I'll typically drink coffee or green tea beforehand. This gives my brain the cognitive boost needed to complete the task successfully.

However, if I'm going out to a restaurant or bar, or I know I'll be walking a lot, I'll typically avoid caffeine to help minimize dyskinesia.

As mentioned earlier, caffeine is known to have neuroprotective effects, but more research is needed to confirm its long-term benefits and whether it helps in slowing the disease progression.

Alcohol

In most cases, PWPs tend to avoid alcohol. There are several reasons for this. First of all, alcohol is often on the banned list for many Parkinson's medications. The reason for this is less about causing liver damage like when mixing alcohol with acetaminophen, and more about the fact that many Parkinson's medications already cause nausea or dizziness; adding alcohol to the mix doesn't help with those symptoms. Another reason to avoid alcohol is that its effects can have a negative impact on your mood and on your ability to move. Alcohol is a downer, which means that for PWPs, our slow movements worsen with alcohol consumption. Over the past several years I have developed a strong negative reaction to alcohol consumption, which could likely be in part due to Parkinson's combined with high blood pressure. I now abstain from consuming alcohol unless it's for a special occasion, and even then, I only drink in moderation.

One interesting finding is that resveratrol, which is found in red wine, has been found to be an excellent antioxidant. However, it's not advised to start drinking a glass of red wine each day just for the resveratrol. Instead, you can purchase resveratrol supplements that have the same efficacy as the real thing but without the alcohol.

Meat

It's a well-known fact that all types of animal meat contain carcinogens and cholesterol, and many are also high in saturated fats. Not only are these elements unhealthy for your heart, but the spread of free radicals can have a negative effect on the health of your brain as well. Red meat is perhaps the most carcinogenic, followed by pork, poultry, then fish. Fish also adds the danger of heavy metal poisoning. While it's not absolutely necessary to completely eliminate all meats from your diet, you certainly want to minimize the amount you eat, perhaps replacing it with plant-based proteins.

Carb / Protein Balance

It's important to have a balance between carbohydrates and protein in your diet, and this is especially true if you are taking carbidopa-levodopa or dopamine agonists. This is because carbidopa-levodopa is best absorbed in the body when taken while your body is digesting carbohydrates. The drug's absorption into the body will be more difficult when your body is processing proteins. This is why some Parkinson's doctors recommend having a diet low in protein and high carbohydrates. In my own experience, I have noticed that plant protein is a lot easier on the digestive system than animal protein. Your body will have less trouble absorbing the medication if you eat proteins like soybeans, legumes, and nuts.

Vitamins C, D, and E

Doctors have increasingly noticed that PWPs are often deficient in vitamins C, D, and E. Vitamins are important for maintaining a healthy immune system, and this is especially important for PWPs. The reason is that we are more likely to get illnesses like aspiration pneumonia, which can lead to hospitalization and could even be fatal. Vitamin C also helps the body heal wounds, which is also helpful since we tend to get more cuts and bruises than most of the general population. The best way to consume vitamin C is, like with all vitamins and minerals, from food. Supplements work fine, but it's best if you get you vitamin C from fresh citrus fruits, tomatoes, and potatoes. Other delicious foods that contain vitamin C include red and green peppers, kiwi, broccoli, strawberries, Brussels sprouts, and cantaloupe.

Vitamin D is a vitamin we naturally receive from the sun, and it helps maintain muscle tone and bone density as we age. However, if you spend many of your days indoors, especially in cooler, rainier, or cloudier climates, you may certainly be deficient in vitamin D. This essential vitamin is linked to mood, and a deficiency could lead to low mood, irritability, and emotional difficulties. We of course want to maintain strong bones as we age because falling and brittle bones do not go well together. As with the other vitamins on this list, it's better to get your required amount with some time in the sun, but you can also use supplements if needed. Besides the sun, get vitamin D from fatty fish, cheese, egg yolk, and fortified milk.

Vitamin E is an important antioxidant that could help prevent the spread of free radicals in the body. It also has immune functions to help keep the body healthy. Most people get their vitamin E from soybean, canola, corn, and other vegetable oils in food products. It's also naturally occurring in nuts, seeds, vegetable oils, as well as in green leafy vegetables and fortified cereals.

Tracking Nutrition

Tracking your nutrition on a daily basis is extremely important in order to understand how each meal affects you and your body. If you are the type of person who tracks calorie intake, that's a good start, but you should also be tracking fat intake, carbohydrates, proteins, and sugars. You'll want to determine what the ideal calorie intake is for someone your age, weight, and height – something your doctor can help you with – and then create a plan to track your food intake to be sure you are within the appropriate range for all of the statistics just mentioned. It may also be useful to check for vitamin deficiencies once a year or so in case anything is below what it should be.

You can combine your nutrition data with your other tracked data to find hills and valleys in the disease progression, and determine if nutrition is playing a positive or negative role. For example, does eating certain fruits or vegetables make you feel more energetic or less so? Each person reacts differently to foods, exercise, and the disease itself, meaning that your tracked data can help you create a personalized plan for yourself.

An easy way to keep track of these items is to use a paper and pen journal or a spreadsheet to keep track of the foods you eat at each meal, including the calorie count. You can keep track of things like fats and sugars as well, but typically it's enough to keep track of what you are eating to keep you thinking actively about your food consumption. What results is a log that we can use to help draw conclusions about how food, medications, and exercise all work together in our overall health. But another reason to keep track of our food intake is to become active in our food consumption process. If we keep track of what we eat, we are more likely to realize when we are overdoing it in certain things like sweets, and we can then adjust our intake in the following days and weeks. Remember, you can't manage what you don't track.

Chapter IX

Medications

Parkinson's disease demands the use of medication. This is an unfortunate fact, and one that every PWP must come to terms with. You may want to put off medications for as long as you can after diagnosis, but after you have reached the limits of the therapeutic effect offered by supplements and natural treatments, we all end up at the pharmacy filling prescriptions for pills we will likely take for the rest of our lives. It does sound pretty sad, but if you are lucky enough to have properly calibrated medications, you will be able to tell the difference and it will make a huge improvement to your life.

There are many different classes of medications for Parkinson's, and since everybody has different symptoms and different severities, no one silver bullet fixes everything. The basic medication for Parkinson's, Sinemet (also called carbidopa-levodopa), is probably the only one that comes close to being a silver bullet, but many PWPs find that this is not enough on its own and most supplement carbidopa-levodopa with other meds over time. Fortunately, there's a vast array of medications for different symptoms, so it's likely that you can find a good mix after discussing it with your medical team and making the appropriate adjustments.

Sinemet

Sinemet is the brand name for carbidopa-levodopa, medication that has been in use for PWPs for decades, and it's seen as the gold standard for use early in the disease. In essence, carbidopa-levodopa is the gateway drug we all start with and that leads us to other, stronger medications. In fact, carbidopa-levodopa can even help with the diagnosis of Parkinson's – you may be prescribed a carbidopa-levodopa trial, and if your symptoms improve, then the diagnosis is most likely Parkinson's.

The way the drug works is simple: levodopa gets converted into dopamine in the brain, so carbidopa-levodopa's job is getting levodopa into your brain. However, the brain has a protective system known as the blood-brain barrier, which evolution has given us as a defense mechanism for the brain, making it nearly impossible for anything to pass through. It makes sense – your brain should be protected from as many external contaminants as possible. To help get the levodopa into the brain so it can become dopamine, it's combined with carbidopa, which helps keep the levodopa from breaking down before it reaches the brain. Think of carbidopa as a cocoon that sacrifices itself to help the levodopa get in. That's one brave little molecule!

Typically, carbidopa and levodopa are paired in a 1-to-4 ratio, so you get pills with 25mg of carbidopa and 100mg of levodopa, or 50mg of carbidopa and 200mg of levodopa. The carbidopa has no therapeutic effect, it's simply there as a way to get the levodopa into the brain. While most people take the instant release version of carbidopa-levodopa with the aim of getting the levodopa into the brain as quickly as possible, some people may take the controlled or extended release version instead of or in addition to the instant release version. The CR or ER variants of carbidopa-levodopa help provide a continuous stream of levodopa over time rather than all at once. The therapeutic effect of carbidopa-levodopa is to make the principle Parkinson's symptoms less apparent or disappear entirely. It's actually quite miraculous to watch someone with tremors, slowness, and stiffness suddenly move freely. Unfortunately, carbidopa-levodopa's ability to provide relief lessens over time and as the disease progresses, but those first few doses seem like magic to the newly-diagnosed PWP.

Carbidopa-levodopa is usually well tolerated, especially in earlier stages of the disease, but there can still be side effects that could be discomforting or even disabling. The most common side effects include nausea and dizziness. Check with your doctor on other side effects, and for things to watch for when taking carbidopa-levodopa. It's safe to say, however, that you should not drive or operate machinery until you know how the medication will affect you. This is also another reason to avoid alcohol while taking it.

Unfortunately, the positive effects of carbidopa-levodopa are reduced over time as the disease progresses. Your body begins to get used to the carbidopa-levodopa and it either stops working altogether, or it has limited effects with more off periods than on, and it introduces new side effects like dyskinesia – uncontrollable body movements. Although there is some controversy regarding when to begin taking carbidopa-levodopa – some believe taking it early in the disease means more time feeling normal, but doing so runs the risk that the medication will stop working sooner, while others want to wait and save the medication until their symptoms become more apparent and disabling. This is open to debate, and is worth discussing with your doctor. Since I was diagnosed at a very young age, I decided to take it right away since it made my symptoms go away and I could continue living a semi-normal life for a few more years. Predictably, after a few years of taking carbidopa-levodopa, the medication is not as effective as it once was.

Dopamine Agonists

Dopamine agonists are likely to be the next step after carbidopa-levodopa has lost its usefulness or has become less effective in controlling motor symptoms. Agonists are available in many different formulations, including in pill form – Requip (also known as ropinerol) and Mirapex (also known as pramipexole), as a subcutaneous continuous injection that can be evenly dispensed throughout the day – Apokyn or Movapo (also known as apomorphine), and as a patch that is put on the patient's arm – Neupro (also known as rotigotine). Nearly everyone I know who uses a dopamine agonist says that they have a love-hate relationship with it. We are about to find out why.

Unlike carbidopa-levodopa, dopamine agonists don't need to be converted into dopamine in the brain. When they are taken, they go straight to the brain and attach themselves directly onto dopamine receptors. In a way, this is a more effective treatment then carbidopa-levodopa, but it doesn't come without its consequences. Some of the more serious side effects of using dopamine agonists include hallucinations, cognitive impairment, and compulsive behaviors. You should discuss with your doctor the pluses and minuses of taking a dopamine agonist, weighing the pros and cons to be sure it's for you. When I was offered dopamine agonists by my neurologist, I declined to take them because my cognition was very good at the time and I didn't want to lose one of the last highly functioning parts of my body. I was also afraid of the more serious side effects.

Let's talk a bit more about the side effect that is considered the big tradeoff of using dopamine agonists: compulsive behaviors. This is one of the most common side effects noted by my Parkinson's friends taking agonists, and I have heard stories about people gambling away their entire life savings, becoming addicted to sex and seeking out the service of prostitutes, or starting to use hard drugs and falling into that deep and scary pit. You know that your Parkinson's has become serious when you're balancing whether the ability to move freely is worth the tradeoff of derailing your life in other ways.

Despite this stern warning that I offer you, I'd recommend discussing dopamine agonists with your doctors to see if they are right for you. They are certainly more effective than carbidopa-levodopa at controlling symptoms, and who doesn't want to have relief from the symptoms of a never-ending disease? Proceed with caution.

Anti-dyskinesia

Carbidopa-levodopa tends to work well in managing symptoms for quite a while, but eventually the medication leads to dyskinesias, which are disabling and often painful excessive movements of the body. To counteract these excessive movements, PWPs are often prescribed Symmetrel (also known as amantadine). This medication often helps in reducing or eliminating levodopa-induced dyskinesia, but even this medication loses its effectiveness over time. Amantadine also causes many side effects, such as constipation, which can lead to other health problems as well. In addition, amantadine cannot be easily stopped during the course of treatment, since this can cause significant side effects like delirium with confusion, disorientation, agitation, and paranoia. If you need to discontinue amantadine, speak to your doctor before doing so.

I began having levodopa-induced dyskinesia starting in early 2014. At the peak effectiveness of my dosing cycle I would experience severe involuntarily movements in my head, neck, shoulders, and especially in my left leg. It got the point where my left leg would kick up uncontrollably whenever I walked, making it difficult to get around even when my medications were on. I began taking amantadine in hopes of reducing or eliminating these dyskinesia, but it only served to slightly reduce the movements in my arms and neck, while the disabling leg movement remained. Over time, the drug did lose its effectiveness in helping to reduce dyskinesia as well. Sometimes I'd take a dose of carbidopa-levodopa without the amantadine to see if it was still helping to reduce dyskinesia – it was helping, but its overall effectiveness had been reduced.

A lesser-known side effect of amantadine, but one that can be scary when it first manifests itself, is the appearance of spots on your arms, legs, and feet. This condition is called livedo reticularis, and although harmless, its appearance could be enough to scare you into a visit to the emergency room. The spots are unsightly and are more likely to appear during colder weather, but the good news is that they disappear when you stop taking amantadine.

MAO-inhibitors

Eldepryl (also known as selegiline) and Azilect (also known as rasagiline), are MAO-inhibiters that can be used in addition to carbidopa-levodopa. They work by increasing the levels of dopamine, norepinephrine, and serotonin in the brain. They can help improve symptoms like shaking, stiffness, and difficulty moving. The side effects of MAO-inhibitors are in some ways similar to those of dopamine agonists – increased compulsivity, hallucinations, and cognitive decline – but also includes other side effects like narcolepsy (falling asleep suddenly and without warning), and sudden jumps in blood pressure, which can be fatal.

As with all the medications we discussed here, it's worth having a conversation with your doctor about your goals for treatment. If you are currently working and use your brain for intense cognitive activities, you may not want to take a medication that could damage cognition. On the other hand, if a job is more physical in nature, you may be okay taking a medication that may cause some cognitive difficulties, though I'd not recommend operating machinery (including driving) while on these medications. When my neurologist recommended I try selegiline, I was worried about its cognitive effects since I had just gone back to school to study business, so I declined her recommendation. Just like with all of the tradeoffs necessary with medications, I had to prioritize what was most important to me – I chose to protect my cognition at the loss of improved movement.

Anti-depressants

There is often controversy surrounding the use of antidepressants in general. It's often said that antidepressants are over-prescribed to treat problems that could be helped through talk therapy. People go on antidepressants for all sorts of reasons: unhappiness at work or in relationships, or because they are simply down about life. It's estimated that 13% of American adults use antidepressants – that is one in every eight American adults. Whatever you feel about the use of antidepressants by the general population, the situation is quite different for PWPs. For us, there is quite literally a chemical imbalance in our brains causing depression, anxiety, and mood changes.

Parkinson's rewires our brains, causing both dopamine and serotonin – chemicals that make us happy – to decrease in our brains.

Although I have incorporated talk therapy into my own wellness routine, with Parkinson's there is no substitute for anti-depressants to battle depression, anxiety, and mood variations. I'd suggest having your neurologist or psychologist refer you to a neuropsychiatrist with experience in treating PWPs to learn more about treatment options.

My neurologist recommended Effexor (also known as venlafaxine), which is a drug in the selective serotonin-norepinephrine reuptake inhibitor (SNRI) class, to combat anxiety and depression. My understanding is that venlafaxine is favored for use with PWPs because it's activating – it acts as a sort of upper that increases serotonin levels in the brain, and it's a drug that fits well with other Parkinson's drugs. In effect, it works well with the changed chemistry in our brains and helps the serotonin do its job. The drug is typically dispensed in 37.5mg capsules, and your doctor will recommend some multiple of this number to indicate how many capsules to take per day. The best part of venlafaxine is its tolerability and its low chance for side effects.

Beta Blockers

Beta blockers are traditionally used to lower blood pressure and to slow the heart. For this reason, they have been banned in most sports because they give athletes an unfair advantage by increasing endurance. While beta blockers find legitimate use with people with heart conditions, surprisingly, beta blockers also work for calming tremors. In fact, beta blockers can be used to treat several conditions simultaneously. There are many different types of beta blockers on the market, but the type that seems to be prescribed often for Parkinson's is the nonselective beta blocker. These include Corgard (also known as nadolol) and Inderal (also known as propranolol).

Long ago, when I first began my Parkinson's journey, I suffered from both high blood pressure – 140/100 was the norm – and from migraines. My left hand had also already begun to show a slight tremor. After speaking with my neurologist, she prescribed nadolol in hopes of working to address all three issues. The result was astounding – my migraines were completely gone, my blood pressure consistently measured 120/80, and my tremor had disappeared (but the slowness and rigidity remained). The only downside to nadolol was that it left me feeling tired and needing a daily afternoon nap. When I moved to Amsterdam, I was told that nadolol was not available so I was switched to propranolol, which made me feel less tired but also brought back a slight tremor in my left hand. There are many different variants of nonselective beta blockers, so it's worth working with your doctor to find the one that works best for you.

Tracking Medications

Tracking your medications is very important, not only for Parkinson's disease, but for any illness. Not taking medications on time as the doctor recommends can lead to anything from a minor inconvenience, to an emergency situation. With some drugs, taking them every day at around the same time is what is recommended. Often, with most drugs if you miss a dose at a specific time, you can just skip that dose and retake it later. This is not the case with Parkinson's medications.

Parkinson's medications have a very short half-life, and they must be taken at the correct times as indicated by your doctor. For example, if your doctor has put you on a schedule of one tablet of carbidopa-levodopa every four hours, taking the medication half an hour early may mean that you have too much levodopa in your brain, causing side effects like dyskinesia. Taking the medication half hour late could mean that there is a gap between doses, which leads to an off period that may last longer than that half-hour between doses, since the carbidopa-levodopa takes some time to build up in your body and become effective after you've taken it. This is why it's so important to keep track of your medications, not only of when you have taken them but also when you should take them next.

Keeping a journal and setting an alarm on your phone for different times could be useful for keeping track of your meds. For me, this became a real hassle because I had to rely on a pen and paper diary that I needed to carry around with me all the time, and setting alarms on my phone using the built-in alarm clock was just too cumbersome for me. My solution was to build a medication tracking system in my app, Parkinson's LifeKit. The app lets me input which medications I take and at what doses, and I can then tell the app to alert me when I need to take a particular medication. Since every day brings different challenges, the app can be told to alert me to take my meds at a particular time of day, or at an interval of time like in 30 minutes or in an hour. This can be useful if you wake up late and need to take a particular medication at an odd time. Once you mark the medications as taken, that dose is stored to your permanent record, which you can review at any time. If you begin feeling some adverse symptom at any point, you can make a note of that as well and let your doctor know next time you see them. Having all of the data in one place makes keeping track of your entire health a lot simpler.

Chapter X

Supplements

Supplements can be a useful part of a PWP's nutritional regimen, since many of us are likely to be deficient in vitamins C, D, and E. We also need higher quantities of neuroprotective acids like Omega-3 than the general population, and the most effective way to get those larger amounts is with supplements. It's important, however, to recognize that the supplement market is full of misinformation and low-quality products that may do more harm than good. Understanding how each supplement is intended to be used, and buying only high quality products from reputable brands are the best ways to ensure you're optimizing your supplement intake.

It may be the case that a naturopathic doctor may have suggested particular supplements for you to take, or perhaps you've read a book about holistic medicine and learned about supplements that might work well for Parkinson's, or maybe you heard it through the grapevine – from a family member or friend – that a particular supplement can help with Parkinson's. I've taken supplements based on the claims and advice from all of these sources, and I have had mixed results. My intention here is to tell you about the science behind these recommendations, and also about the anecdotal evidence that exists, which is not always to be fully trusted. By focusing on the science rather than solely on anecdotal evidence, we can ensure that we're not wasting our time, money, and energy on supplements that provide false hope.

A Few Words About Supplements and Science

At this point, I should point out some important critical thinking skills that all PWPs need to learn in order to avoid disappointment. Since we're stricken with a debilitating, incurable disease, we're likely targets of dishonest people trying to sell us things that they say will give us relief but really will not. Unfortunately, the idea of snake oil – a product that doesn't do what it's advertised to do – still exists, and people are out there ready to prey on your emotions and take your money. I have seen this dozens of times, and now the internet makes it easier than ever to make a wild claim that some "ancient herb" or "leaf consumed for centuries" may help either treat or cure Parkinson's.

Let me make this absolutely clear: at this time, there is no cure for Parkinson's disease. There is no herb, vitamin, mineral, therapy, pill, or device that has been scientifically proven to stop, delay, or reverse the disease's progression. If such a thing existed, I guarantee you that everybody would know about it – It would be on the front page of every major newspaper in the world. The only thing that has actually been scientifically proven to slow the progression is exercise.

With that said, anybody who claims to have a cure for Parkinson's, and they advertise that on their website complete with testimonials and a research study, is lying to you and manipulating you in some way. I have seen every type of scam, including having acupuncture needles implanted into your earlobes, taking a special supplement that is suspiciously only available from a single pharmacy in the whole world, and even people saying they will coach you into being cured of Parkinson's. I'll not hesitate to proclaim that none of these things will cure Parkinson's.

Please do your own research for anything you decide to put into your body, or anytime you decide to pay someone for something. Find out if there is reputable research behind it, which typically means finding research that is corroborated by even more research behind it. A single study is usually not enough to tell you if something works or not. In my own examination of supplements and alternative therapies, I'll tell you that most outcomes and positive experiences are anecdotal – passed on from patient to patient – but are not backed by science. I will not be discussing supplements that I've tried or heard about and which I know are based on pseudoscience or fake science. I'll only discuss supplements I have tried and/or which have been studied scientifically and verified as effective as general supplements, but not necessarily specific only to Parkinson's. In other words, these supplements may be useful to take to promote general good health, but they may one day be proven to help specifically with parts of the brain affected by Parkinson's, as is the case with antioxidants.

Ultimately, the main point here is patient beware. There are a lot of shady people out there ready to prey on your fears and desperation for a few bucks. Do your own research on everything and learn to tell what is scientific fact and what is snake oil.

Vitamin C – 3,000mg

Vitamin C is a powerful antioxidant, and has been used for many years as a way to boost the immune system. It's best to get vitamin C from natural foods like citrus fruits (oranges, grapefruits), but it's possible to get your vitamin C from supplements as well. When possible, and as with all supplements, try to get the vitamin C tablets or capsules that contain the least amount of fillers. The typical dose commonly recommended for a healthy adult is about 1,000mg per day. For PWPs, I have heard of doctors who recommend taking as much as 3,000mg per day as a form of neuroprotection. As a bonus, vitamin C will help protect against colds.

Resveratrol – 100mg

Resveratrol is a known antioxidant that is naturally found in red wine. If you already drink red wine regularly, then you are likely already benefiting from this neuroprotective chemical. However, I would not recommend starting to drink red wine just for the benefits of resveratrol. The recommended way of getting this antioxidant for a PWP is in capsule form, since drinking alcohol is contraindicative to the disease. Resveratrol provides a similar effect to vitamin C, so if you are already taking one, you will not necessarily need to take both.

Vitamin D – 400-1,000IU

Vitamin D naturally comes from the sun, and is something we all need. Vitamin D plays a role in cellular and brain health, since our neurons have vitamin D receptors that need to be nourished. As important as vitamin D is for general good health, vitamin D deficiency is quite common among PWPs. This is especially problematic because vitamin D also contributes to bone health, and PWPs need strong bones to withstand falls. Brittle bones combined with poor balance can lead to devastating falls, which could lead to complications and death. Not to put too fine a point on it, but PWPs need vitamin D and being deficient is a high risk none of us should take.

If you are the type of person who doesn't get enough sun, either because you do not go outside often or because you live in a place that lacks constant sunshine, then most doctors would recommend taking a vitamin D supplement. Living in Seattle, I was told by every doctor that I needed to take vitamin D supplements. My naturopath recommended 1,000IUs (international units), but check with your doctor before starting on your own vitamin D regimen.

Green Tea Extract – 500mcg

Green tea has been used as a mood enhancer, as well as an antioxidant. One cup of green tea per day is enough to get your body and mind going. If you are not much of a tea drinker, you can also find green tea extract in powder or capsule form. If you get the capsules, you can take them in the morning along with your regular medications and they should provide you with increased mental agility and improved movement. One thing to beware of: green tea contains caffeine, certainly less than in coffee, but be aware of this in case you already consume caffeine from coffee as part of your daily routine. There is such a thing as too much caffeine, so you may want to pull back on the coffee if you decide to add green tea or a green tea supplement to your routine.

Curcumin

Curcumin is an Indian spice that surprisingly also has neuroprotective qualities. It's available in powder form, and its power, although anecdotal for the most part, is such that it can protect the neurons of people suffering from many chronic neurological conditions. Doctors have told me to buy curcumin in its powder form at a supermarket and mix it into the foods I cook on a daily basis. What I like best about curcumin is that it's a natural spice and is sold in its raw form, free of the manipulation and processing of commercial supplements. This means that you're not taking yet another pill, and if science later discovers that curcumin is not really that useful for neuroprotection, at least it's delicious and natural!

Creatine

Creatine is a natural compound that plays an important role in the way our cells get their energy. It's an antioxidant that shows promise to help "clean out" the accumulation of free radicals that lead to peripheral nerve damage. Creatine has been extensively studied for its potential benefits for Parkinson's, but results are mixed. A recent meta-analysis, the analysis of multiple piece of research to get a better idea of creatine's potential, showed that while some research indicated that creatine could help delay Parkinson's progression, other research has shown that it doesn't do anything compared to placebo. The authors of the study concluded that more research is needed, so be aware that there is no conclusive scientific evidence behind the assertion that creatine is helpful to delay Parkinson's.

Coenzyme Q10

CoQ10, as it's commonly referred to, is an antioxidant that was previously thought to be beneficial for slowing the disease progression by supporting cellular function. In theory, this sounds like it should work, but past studies have been mixed regarding CoQ10's effectiveness. When I was first diagnosed, my movement disorder specialist recommended I take CoQ10 as a way to delay the progression. More recently, the research has shown that it actually shows no benefit compared to placebo. In other words, it doesn't do what we had hoped it would do. If someone suggests you take CoQ10 as a way of delaying Parkinson's progression, I recommend you first take a look at the 2014 paper by the Parkinson Study Group to review their research (link in the appendix).

Omega-3 Fatty Acid

Omega-3 fatty acids are among some of the best-known substances to help alleviate Parkinson's symptoms naturally. While it's best to get your omega-3 fatty acids from actual fish, buying a well-produced and natural fatty acid supplement with verified ingredients can be just as good as the real thing. Omega-3 fatty acids are capable of crossing the blood-brain barrier, unlike most other supplements and medications, since the body's own defense system stops this from happening. When the fatty acids get into the brain, they can increase blood flow and reduce neural inflammation in the brain. In addition, Omega-3 has been shown to help restore some cognitive dysfunction like memory loss. Omega-3 contains an acid that has been shown to reduce motor symptoms and inflammation in animal models. In your own research, you may find that many of the studies about Omega-3 have been conducted using placebo amounts of EPA, which didn't show significant results. You may want to exclude those studies from your own research and instead focus on studies that use full-strength Omega-3 acids, like those contained in commercially available capsules.

Tracking Supplements

Tracking supplements is of particular importance due to the fact that there is so little research behind the claims made by many supplement proponents. A certain supplement may work effectively in just a few small studies, while longer-range and broader studies might show that there really is no benefit after all. Tracking your use of supplements can help determine whether certain supplements work for you or not. This is especially true with PWPs, since we often experience a placebo effect when we begin taking a new supplement or drug.

Some research has shown that when PWPs begin taking a new medication or supplement, the first few doses give us a boost of dopamine and serotonin, making us believe that the new treatment is working. It's not until a week or two into the new treatment that we realize whether the new treatment is effective. At first, we're excited about the prospects of the new treatment, but after our dopamine levels go back to normal, the treatment will show a positive effect or it won't. This is why longer-range studies are so important.

You can use a diary, spreadsheet, or the Parkinson's LifeKit app to track your supplements. It's useful to not only track supplements, but also other factors like physical, cognitive, and emotional fitness. This will help you discover connections between a supplement and your overall health. If after a week, you believe a supplement is helping you physically, great. But how does it perform over a month or six months? That is the real test to whether a supplement is truly useful or not.

Another suggestion when tracking supplements is to start or stop only one particular supplement at a time. If your doctor says, "you should take X, Y, and Z," first try X by itself to see if you benefit from X. Then perhaps a few months later you can add Y and see if you notice an improvement. Finally, after a few more months you can start Z and see how your body reacts to that change. Only by introducing (or removing) one supplement at a time, and tracking your fitness and symptoms over time, will you be able to tell which supplements are actually working and which are not. You can also remove supplements this same way to determine if a supplement is negatively affecting your health.

As you can see there are many variables to consider when taking supplements. The important thing is to see what works for you, and then eliminate what doesn't work for you. Remember, everyone is different and will react differently to different supplements. Since there is still much research to be done on supplements, it's important to follow the research and reassess when new research is released. I'd also recommend asking your doctors which brands they recommend, but beware of doctors (especially naturopaths) who only recommend brands that they carry at their practice and that they want you to buy. Oftentimes the naturopath will tell you they carry and recommend a certain brand because of its superior quality, however in most cases the supplements your doctor is selling was manufactured by a company also selling it online with a different label and for less money. Always buy your supplements from a reputable store that is independent of your doctor's business.

Chapter XI

Medical Marijuana

With new laws allowing the use of medical and recreational marijuana throughout the United States and around the world, the use of marijuana as a treatment for Parkinson's has gotten a lot of attention lately. Unfortunately, since it's so new and since there isn't enough research available as of yet, there are a lot of misunderstandings about what medical marijuana is, and how it can help with the symptoms of Parkinson's disease. I have had some experience in the research of medical marijuana, and for the sake of completeness, I want offer some views, some colloquial experience results, and point you towards research currently being done in the field.

Western Views

As I mentioned, medical marijuana has not been studied thoroughly, and so there is not much scientific research available to test the claims that proponents make. In the United States, federally-funded research into the benefits of medical marijuana is non-existent because marijuana is listed as a Schedule I drug by the Drug Enforcement Administration. This puts marijuana on the same level as LSD, ecstasy, heroin, and meth. Any research that has been conducted about marijuana was focused on its negative effects rather than on discovering its benefits. Researchers will obviously only find bad things to say about marijuana if their research questions are something like, "how bad is marijuana...," rather than asking, "can marijuana help with tremors?" The doctors I have spoken with regarding the use of medical marijuana have told me to stay away from it. This is predictable, since licensed doctors could get into trouble for recommending the use of an illegal narcotic. My neurologist also told me that marijuana is contraindicated for Parkinson's, meaning that marijuana could worsen my symptoms.

I believe there are two reasons why traditional doctors will not prescribe or even recommend marijuana for Parkinson's. First, as I have already mentioned, doctors could get into trouble for recommending or likely even suggesting the use of marijuana to treat symptoms. They do not want to get sued by patients if something goes wrong, and they don't want to lose their medical licenses for recommending the use of an illegal drug. The second reason why traditional doctors will want to stay away from medical marijuana is because it's not properly understood by science, and as scientists, they would not want to be involved with anything that has not been thoroughly studied for safety and efficacy.

Doctors frequently refer to marijuana as a single drug and with a single effect on the body. For example, they hear "marijuana" and they instantly think about teenagers getting high, having bloodshot eyes, and smoking for recreational use. They fail to recognize the fact that marijuana is as complex a crop as grapes, for example. You would not say that there is only one type of grape with one single flavor, would you? The same is true for marijuana. There are different strains and different parts of the plant that have different effects on the body. So to make a blanket statement about marijuana would be incorrect.

There are two main strains of marijuana plants – the Indica strain, which provides a body high, could be seen as contraindicated for Parkinson's because it's a downer – people who use Indica-dominant marijuana find it easier to be relaxed and get to sleep. However, marijuana from the Sativa strain provides more of a head high, making you feel uplifted and energized. Sativa-dominant marijuana could actually help improve mood and mobility since it's an upper. Both Indica and Sativa marijuana variants get their psychoactive ingredients from a chemical in the plant called THC. The higher the THC in the marijuana, the stronger the effect (downer for Indica, upper for Sativa) will be.

It's very important to note, however, that there is a part of the marijuana plant that contains only the cannabinoids and doesn't contain the psychoactive ingredient THC, and is typically referred to as CBD. CBD can be made into oils that you can take with a dropper or in capsule form. CBD is what many in the medical marijuana community are referring to when they talk about marijuana for medicinal purposes. The end product of a CBD oil can be made to contain no THC at all. This means that you could take CBD capsules as medicine and not get a high. Let me repeat this because it's critical: CBD oil capsules and drops can be made to contain no psychoactive effects because CBD doesn't contain THC.

Proponents of CBD claim that it can be used to fight pain, and as we will soon learn, many in the Parkinson's community are excited for its potential uses in treating tremors and dyskinesia. CBD has even been used to treat a child with seizures. She became so famous from her experience that the strain she used was named after her, and now Charlotte's Web is one of the most sought after varietals in the medical marijuana community.

If you are fortunate enough to live in a state or country that allows the use of medical marijuana, I highly recommend speaking to a naturopathic doctor about your options. The doctor can recommend the use of marijuana for treating Parkinson's, suggest what specific varietals or brand names to look for, and can also help adjust your diet and exercise routine as well. In my state of Washington, where both medical and recreational marijuana are legal, I was able to visit a naturopath who gave me advice on what to use for Parkinson's symptoms. I was surprised how professional the dispensaries and products appeared. In Washington State, Marijuana is highly regulated, so each product is tested for purity, level of THC or CBD, and quality. The packaging of each product clearly states strain, varietal, percentage of THC and/or CBD, date of harvest, and much more. This is a much different experience than in Amsterdam, where I think even the people selling the marijuana don't know exactly what they're selling. It's important to find reputable vendors, just as you would when selecting supplement brands.

A Short Intro

I want to describe a bit about the different strains and potencies of medical marijuana, especially as it has been used by many people in the Parkinson's community to treat specific symptoms related to the disease. Like I said, there hasn't been much research done regarding marijuana for Parkinson's, but colloquially there have been some stories and experiences that are worth sharing.

Learning about marijuana for use with Parkinson's can be a daunting task, and it can also be embarrassing to go into one of these stores and ask for specific strains by name, since the producers of these products don't do us any favors by naming them strange things like Alice in Wonderland,

Super Silver Haze, and AK-47. Some names are even stranger than that, since the primary target market for these products are people in their 20s.

A note about smoking marijuana versus ingesting it in other forms: Traditionally, those using marijuana as a recreational drug have smoked it out of a pipe or as a pre-roll (aka, a joint). I don't condone smoking anything, since this can lead to other serious health problems like lung cancer. If you are going to use marijuana, I recommend buying oil-based tinctures or capsules, although the response time is slow since it must go through your digestive system. For a faster response you may also look into using a vaporizer, which burns marijuana like when using a pipe, but which only produces vapor as its output.

Battling Pain

Pain is something that we deal with when we have Parkinson's. I've definitely experienced pain from poor posture and bad walking form. I have dealt with lower back pain, hip pain, and muscle aches. I'd typically medicate the pains with ibuprofen or acetaminophen, but neither of these drugs offer a long-term solution due to their side effects. Many people are rightly concerned with eventual liver damage or damage to the stomach lining when taking traditional painkillers over many years. It would be great if a more natural method of treating chronic pain existed.

Medical marijuana derived from the plant's cannabinoids excels at reducing and even eliminating pain. It acts directly on to the pain receptors in the brain and numbs them to pain. Several people in the Seattle Parkinson's community have told me that smoking Charlotte's Web takes pain away in minutes while a more gradual CBD capsule takes a little longer to take effect but they provide for extended pain relief.

Battling Depression

Depression is something many of us with Parkinson's face on a regular basis. This depression comes from a chemical deficiency in our brains, in which dopamine and serotonin – two chemicals that contribute to an uplifted mood – are reduced. This chemical imbalance can be helped by replacing the dopamine with medications, such as by using carbidopa-levodopa, but this is typically not enough to do the job. Sativa-based medical marijuana that is high in THC has been used to improve mood, increase focus and concentration, and generally enhance mental state.

Keep in mind that THC is a psychoactive ingredient that acts on the dopamine receptors in the brain. Those who are early in the disease may need less to lift their mood than those who are further along. I have found that the later in the disease you are, the fewer dopamine receptors working in your brain, the more of the drug you need to have an effect. I have heard and read anecdotes that 0.5g of high-THC sativa-dominant marijuana can lift moods for several hours. Since THC is a psychoactive, it can cause similar effects on the body as alcohol. Don't drive a vehicle or operate machinery while using this medication.

Some strains to research further are Alice in Wonderland, Super Green Crack, Hawaiian Punch, or Pineapple Super Silver Haze. Remember that marijuana strains are named to appeal to young people, thus these strange names. I believe that once medical marijuana becomes legitimized through extensive scientific research, the most medically significant strains will be renamed to something more dignified. As usual, do your own research and visit with a licensed naturopathic doctor before using any of these medical marijuana products. The website Leafly.com contains comprehensive data on every popular strain in the United States, including uses and side effects – this may make for a great starting point in your research.

Tremors and Dyskinesia

In the past few years, I have watched videos on YouTube and have read discussions in online forums in which PWPs have been sharing their stories of using medical marijuana to treat tremors and dyskinesia. In my personal experience and in my own research, I have found some anecdotal evidence that CBD oil or pure leaf marijuana with a 100-to-1 CBD ratio may help reduce tremors. Others have been inspired by these videos and online discussions, went out and tried CBD for tremors, and they had no reduction in tremor at all. I have not found much evidence, even anecdotal, that CBD oil works for dyskinesia. Again, these are just stories from people sharing their unscientific experiences to the Parkinson's community. Just like with supplements or medications, I suggest you work closely with a naturopathic doctor and try a variety of strains and delivery methods to find out if any of these medications help alleviate your symptoms.

More Research Needed

I truly believe that medical marijuana could become a key part of a PWP's overall treatment, however, much more research needs to be done before that can be the case. In addition, marijuana must be legalized, at minimum for medicinal purposes. Medicinal use cases have shown early promise, and with proper regulation of quality standards, medical marijuana can be life-changing for people living with Parkinson's. I believe that when marijuana is well-researched and accepted as a real medication, it could be a safe and natural replacement for commercial painkillers. It seems that there are advances every day in this respect, but it will take some time until we get to that point.

Chapter XII

Advanced Therapies

When traditional medications are no longer working as intended it may be worth looking into these advanced therapies. I call them advanced for two reasons. First, these are therapies you typically only consider when you have exhausted all medication option, and your symptoms are severely impacting your quality of life. Second, we call these advanced therapies because they are invasive, requiring surgery and implanting devices to help regulate Parkinson's symptoms. Many people who choose these therapies have done so after a long process in which they have weighed the dangers of surgery with the possibilities of having a better quality of life for more years.

DBS

Deep brain stimulation, or DBS, is a neurosurgical procedure that involves implanting a neuro-stimulator (like a pacemaker for the brain) that controls electrodes implanted into specific targets in the brain. The electrical signals sent to the brain serve to short-circuit the brain's Parkinson's activity. The result is a reduction or even elimination of certain motor symptoms such as tremor, slow movement, and rigidity. In many cases, DBS could also help patients reduce their Parkinson's medications, resulting in fewer side effects like dyskinesia. DBS is not a cure for Parkinson's, as the disease still progresses and adjustments need to be made over time, but it's as close to a miracle therapy that we have.

There is a lot to know about DBS, and it's worth finding information online from a hospital that performs the procedure, but I'd like to provide you with some basics to get you started.

DBS has traditionally been known as a therapy of last resort for many patients, submitting themselves to brain surgery when their medications are no longer working like they are supposed to. However, recently DBS has started being used earlier and earlier in the disease, since research has shown positive outcomes for those who get it sooner rather than wait until later when few options remain. DBS has also become more popular with those diagnosed with young-onset Parkinson's, since it can allow them to return to work and also continue many of their favorite activities. Up until recently, one company dominated the DBS hardware market in the United States: Medtronic. However, now there are more companies entering the marketplace including Abbott (St. Jude Medical) and Boston Scientific. Thanks to the increased competition, DBS is now advancing and new and exciting innovations are on the horizon. For example, the new devices have rechargeable batteries that can last a decade or more (minimizing the number of future battery-replacement surgeries), and the new electrode leads are thinner and can more finely target areas in the brain to help minimize side effects.

We know that DBS is not for everyone. Hospitals that perform the procedure put potential patients through a battery of tests, physical, cognitive, emotional, and so on. A good candidate is someone who is far enough along in their disease for their medications to have stopped working like they are supposed to, but not to the point where an intensive surgery would be unsafe. You must also have a response to carbidopa-levodopa, even if that medication no longer works properly for you, since DBS acts in your brain as if the area that controls movement was medicated with carbidopa-levodopa. If you are a good candidate for DBS, having surgery may allow you to return to work and spend more time doing the things you love. Seeing is believing, so to see how DBS has changed the lives of thousands of PWPs, search YouTube for DBS videos. There are several in which the PWP turns off the stimulator momentarily to show their untreated Parkinson's symptoms, and then turns it back on for comparison. It truly seems miraculous.

The one thing that creates fear in people's minds, and is likely to be the reason that DBS is still underutilized around the world, is that this is delicate brain surgery. There is a small chance, probably 1% to 3%, that some complication can occur. Complications can be as small as an infection, which can be prevented quite easily and is considered the PWP's responsibility after they leave the hospital. The worst-case scenarios are aneurysm, stroke, and even death, all of which could occur during surgery. These outcomes are extremely rare, and none of the dozens of surgeons around the US west coast and in Europe I have talked to have had any fatalities, but this is worth mentioning. When you visit a neurosurgery facility to discuss DBS with their staff, it's important to ask about their complication rates. They will tell you exactly what kinds of complications they have seen, how many of each, and the severity of the complications. One neurosurgeon I spoke with in Europe told me that of the thousands of patients he has operated on over the years, two had infections after surgery, and only one had an aneurism. That's a complication rate of around 0.1% - an amazingly low number that should inspire confidence.

Another thing that probably prevents many people from having this procedure done is the fact that it's a major operation, and there are times during the operation in which the patient must be awake. This can be extremely frightening for the patient! Luckily, this is starting to change and many facilities are beginning to offer asleep DBS in which you are under general anesthesia during the entire procedure Depending on several factors, including the hospital, the surgeon, the type of operation, and the hardware being used, asleep DBS may or may not be an option. Awake DBS can be physically strenuous and is not recommended if you are an anxious person. It can be scary to have your head inside a metallic cage in which you cannot move and where doctors are working behind you on your brain. However, from the people I have spoken with, there is no pain during the awake surgery, and the most exciting moment is when they test the implanted lead and your Parkinson's symptoms suddenly disappear. Once the surgeon has properly placed the lead, the patient is put under general anesthesia for the remainder of the procedure. You then awaken in the recovery room with bandages on your head and (outside of the US) the stimulator under your skin below your collarbone. In the US, most insurance companies don't pay for the stimulator to be implanted on the same day as the electrodes, so the PWP must return a couple of weeks later to implant the stimulator.

I would certainly recommend researching DBS, especially if you feel you may be a good candidate for the procedure. Only one person I have spoken to out of a several hundred people with DBS say they would not do it again. The overwhelming majority of PWPs with DBS say they would do it again in a heartbeat; most have said the surgery has given them their lives back. If you are in a country that has approved the new devices by Abbott (St. Jude Medical) and Boston Scientific, I recommend researching those devices in addition to those by Medtronic. Some facilities work with only one brand – usually Medtronic – while others work with Medtronic and another brand, and a few even support all three.

Duopa Pump

If brain surgery sounds a bit too scary and you would like to try other advanced therapies first, a Duopa pump could be the answer. A tube is inserted into the PWP's stomach so that a steady stream of carbidopa-levodopa can be delivered continuously throughout the day. This is a much more efficient way of delivering levodopa to the body, since it bypasses the lengthy digestion process of taking a pill, and allow the medication to reach the brain much more consistently. This is a useful therapy if carbidopa-levodopa still works fairly well for you, but you're experiencing unpredictable or inconsistent on-off periods. While the surgery for this therapy is perhaps seen as being safer than brain surgery, it's not without its own risks. Infection is still a possibility, not only during surgery but after surgery as well, since you are dealing with a sensitive opening in the stomach that is susceptible to bacteria.

This a valid option for those who would want to delay brain surgery, but whose drugs are still working relatively as they should. The digestive system is where the medication's molecules break down and begin coursing through the body, so by injecting the medication straight into the stomach, the Duopa pump bypasses the digestive system and allows the medication to be absorbed directly into the body. The surgery, however, is not useful if your medications have stopped working as they should. In my own case, I was not a candidate for this type of pump because my medications had become ineffective in maintaining my on and off periods throughout the day –

every on stage was accompanied by dyskinesia, and every off stage was accompanied by extreme bradykinesia. This meant that any amount of carbidopa-levodopa entering my system would prove ineffective in properly treating my symptoms.

Chapter XIII

What Does the Future Hold?

The biggest word in the Parkinson's community is "hope." Without a cure, all we can do as PWPs facing the Ballsy Palsy is hope that a cure or disease-modifying therapy comes along sooner than later. There is a lot of ongoing research that gives life to the hope we feel, and new and improved non-cure therapies are released every year, improving our lives while we wait for the big day when we can eliminate the Parkinson's from our bodies for good. Here are some areas in therapy development that should have us excited and hopeful.

New Drug Delivery Methods

Many of the new therapies being released recently are versions of older medications with new delivery methods. For example, although carbidopa-levodopa exists in a long release form, many people do not digest those tablets very well and so the intended delayed release would not happen as intended. That is when a drug company developed and released a drug called Rytary, which is a capsule containing many tiny capsules of carbidopa-levodopa that dissolve at different intervals. This is quite brilliant in many ways. Medically, it's brilliant because it takes medication that already exists and is proven to be safe (helping to avoid costly and lengthy early-stage drug trials), and it's made to be more effective in the patient's body. The medication does this by making the tiny capsules inside dissolve at different times. Some of the tiny capsules dissolve immediately, while others take a few hours to dissolve. The dose is so small in each tiny capsule that one capsule of Rytary releases much less carbidopa-levodopa than a regular tablet. Doctors therefore prescribe a higher dosage of Rytary than what someone would take as a regular instant-release tablet, since the full effect of a Rytary will be felt over a longer period of time.

Another medication that is being re-packaged in a new delivery method is apomorphine. This dopamine agonist is usually available as a pill or as a subcutaneous injection, but it's now being developed in the form of a dissolving sheet that slips under your tongue, similar to the breath strips created years ago to help improve breath by dissolving one on your tongue. The goal is to give patients a quick pick-me-up between doses, or to make up for a skipped dose of other medications. When the patient feels that their medications have worn off unexpectedly, they simply place a breath strip under their tongue, then wait a minute while it dissolves. Ideally, the on-effect arrives within ten minutes. This is another brilliant use of existing medication redesigned to work in a new and more effective way. I participated in a clinical trial to test the effectiveness of these apomorphine breath strips, but they were not very effective in my case because of my issues with dyskinesia.

Nicotine

Nicotine is a chemical gaining in interest with researchers in the Parkinson's community. Early studies and anecdotal evidence show that nicotine, not tobacco or cigarettes but nicotine itself as a pure chemical, can actually help calm dyskinesias. This is somewhat controversial because when we think nicotine we automatically think tobacco and cigarettes; however, this is not that. People doing the research studies use vapes with pure nicotine juices that don't contain any tobacco, poisons, or artificial ingredients. The vapes also don't create any smoke, and the user is only inhaling pure vapor. Of course, as PWPs we don't need another thing to worry about like lung cancer, so using pure vapor is the safest way to ingest nicotine.

After speaking with people involved in advocating for studies with nicotine, I decided to try vaping nicotine myself to see if it would calm my dyskinesias. In fact, I did have success with this technique. Nicotine for vaping is sold in 3mg increments from 3mg to 18mg, and it's available in juice form and in lots of different flavors from lots of different brands. When shopping for nicotine vape juice, you'll want to pick a brand that doesn't use artificial ingredients, as some do. I started vaping with 3mg nicotine juice, and while I did notice some calming of my dyskinesias, I realized that it could be more effective if I increased the dosage. A month after starting on 3 mg, I increased my dosage to the other end of the spectrum – 18 mg. I noticed that this did calm my dyskinesias, but it also made me feel light-headed and dizzy. The sweet spot for me is somewhere in the middle, probably around 9 mg.

We are just at the beginning stages of using nicotine as a way to calm dyskinesia. A lot more research needs to be done with the use of nicotine, not to mention educating the public about the difference between vaping with pure nicotine and smoking cigarettes. However, early indications show promise for nicotine, and I look forward to reading more research about it in the coming years. For now, I'd suggest searching Google or YouTube for information and videos about using nicotine for Parkinson's. Also, this is too cutting edge for most doctors to know much about it, let alone give you the go-ahead to try this yourself. Proceed with caution, and keep an eye on the research.

Stem Cells

Stem cells can be described as universal cells that can be made into any other cell in the body. This holds promise for Parkinson's because of the possibility of converting stem cells into dopamine-producing cells in the brain. In the late 1990s and early 2000s there was much excitement about stem cells with a lot of early-stage research. Much of that excitement went away after the Bush administration slowed and eventually stopped research on stem cells due to ethical issues regarding how they were harvested. While this stopped the research for almost a decade, some progress was made. Experiments were done, and although certain early signs were positive, there are still problems with the technique. Specifically, it seemed that whenever stem cells were implanted into the patient, the cells would gravitate towards becoming cancer cells, which is a huge problem. Specifically, in its use for Parkinson's, newly created neurons would cause dyskinesia in the patient, similar to the effect of long-term carbidopa-levodopa use. Today, scientists have learned how to create stem cells of good quality that are ethically harvested, in fact, coming from the patient's own body. This advance in stem cell science has helped bring new interest to stem cell therapy as a potential cure, or at least as a therapy, in the near future.

Gene Therapy & CRISPR

On the extreme cutting-edge of the therapy spectrum, is gene editing and CRISPR. This technology has the potential to revolutionize medicine, and it's the subject of a lot of controversy, even while still in its infancy. Gene editing involves extracting a piece of DNA from a patient, editing a particular gene – turning something on or off – and then injecting the patient with a DNA virus of sorts, causing the eventual change of all the DNA in the patient's body. Beyond the ethical dilemmas of changing genes of fetuses in-utero and making mosquitos go extinct by turning off their reproductive systems, this technology holds a lot of promise for Parkinson's. Scientists are discovering that genes could play a larger role in Parkinson's than previously thought. For example, we know that the LRRK2 gene plays a role, but there may be others as well. Imagine being able to "fix" the genetic mutation that causes and progresses Parkinson's. You could arrive to the clinic in the morning, have your genes edited in the afternoon, and in a couple of days you would be free of Parkinson's. It sounds like science fiction, and it sounds too good to be true, but this technology is real, albeit still in early stages. Ready to be amazed? Search YouTube for videos about the editing technology, CRISPR, and see what is already being done in this field even today.

Low-Dose Naltrexone (LDN), A Cautionary Tale

Low Dose Naltrexone, or LDN as it's commonly known, was a quasi-naturopathic drug I had read about online. Upon further research, I discovered that several naturopaths in my area had been studying it for its supposed benefits for Parkinson's. Naltrexone itself is a medication aimed at helping people with alcohol and opioid dependencies. In Parkinson's, the drug is actually used as a way to curb the compulsive tendencies that come with taking dopamine agonists. LDN is a low-dose form of Naltrexone, and when taken at bedtime, is supposed to help with symptoms like tremor and stiffness.

After visiting a famous Parkinson's-focused naturopath in the Seattle area, she recommended trying LDN to see if it would help my symptoms. This was before I had started taking carbidopa-levodopa, during the time I had been experimenting with supplements and other natural remedies to avoid taking strong prescription medications. This was in 2012, when many still believed that starting with prescription medications like carbidopa-levodopa later in the disease would extend the amount of time that these drugs would be useful. Today, it's believed that starting prescription medications early after diagnosis has no negative effect, and it would certainly improve quality of life. I was willing to try anything natural before going to pharmaceuticals, so that's a big reason I decided to give LDN a try.

In order to get the correct dosing, I'd have to go to a compounding pharmacy, since LDN was not available anywhere as a readily-available over-the-counter medication. I took my prescription to a compounding pharmacy in my area in the east side of Seattle, and they were able to fill my prescription of LDN in just a couple of days. The instructions were to take one pill at bedtime every night. I was told not to expect immediate results, and reading online, I saw that it took quite a while to feel the therapeutic effect. I gave this therapy six months. In the end, I had not been helped at all by LDN, and without prescription drugs, my quality of life suffered during this time.

My story of using LDN is a perfect example of pseudoscience at work. After LDN provided me no relief, I went back to Google and searched for reputable scientific studies that showed a benefit of using LDN to alleviate Parkinson's symptoms; I found no such study. Websites that claim that LDN works are usually connected to someone selling a book or someone selling LDN online. This experience turned out to be a valuable learning experience for me. I realized that there are people out there who are willing to sell cures and remedies to people looking for these cures and remedies, even though what they are selling is useless.

Experimental Therapy: Glutathione Inhaler

Glutathione is a chemical produced by the body to fuel dopamine-producing cells. PWPs are known to have Glutathione deficiencies, and so one naturopath studied the effects of delivering Glutathione nasally to help treat Parkinson's. The therapy, which is still experimental, uses a Glutathione inhaler to send a shot of the chemical straight to the brain by way of the sinuses. In theory, replacing the brain's Glutathione should provide a therapeutic effect. My Parkinson's naturopath suggested I conduct a trial of intranasal Glutathione as a part of research she was doing. I was skeptical that this would work, but as a PWP desperate for relief from symptoms, I decided to give it a try. There was only one pharmacy in my region that sold glutathione in an inhaler – according to the naturopath, Glutathione is difficult to stabilize in this form, and this was the only pharmacy to have done it successfully.

After two months of using the inhaler daily, shooting the cold liquid up my nostrils and waiting for a result, I didn't experience any alleviation of symptoms. I was told that I may see some relief if I continued using the inhaler for many more months, but this would have been an expensive proposition – I seem to remember it costing about $150 monthly) – and one that didn't provide any clear benefit, so I stopped taking it. While I'm not ready to rule this out as a viable therapy, more scientific research needs to be done by reputable third parties not connected to any pharmacy.

New Research on the Horizon

Although we still don't have a cure, and our best treatment is still the same pill that was used to treat Parkinson's 50 years ago, there is new research on the horizon. I constantly read about different studies and research happening around the world. My desire to always be up-to-date with the latest Parkinson's news lead me to launch Parkinson's Warrior, a resource portal at https://parkinsonswarrior.com. One of the main resources is an aggregated Parkinson's news feed, where you can read the latest research and stories from the community from around the world. From what I read every week, I'm optimistic that we are nearing a cure. Some of the most exciting research I read about involves the use of animal models – using lab mice to test new theories and techniques. Unfortunately, many of the animal models don't translate well into humans, but those that do can show some real promise.

There are reasons to be optimistic. Some recent discoveries include a cancer drug that might help fight Parkinson's, research showing that Parkinson's may originate in the gut, which may lead to new treatments, and that certain foods could help prevent or delay the disease. There are dozens of scientific studies going on at any time, not to mention the numerous drug trials and the human trials for new procedures and therapies.

Get Involved in Clinical Studies!

If you want to be involved in helping to find a cure for Parkinson's, the best way to do that is to get involved in clinical studies. There are always studies looking for new participants, and you might be involved in anything from tracking your fitness every day and reporting that back to the doctors of the study, to taking a new type of medication that has just been approved for human trials. Not only are these trials looking for people at different stages of Parkinson's, but they're also looking for healthy control subjects as well. This is a great opportunity to have your friends and family be involved in the process.

Clinical trials are always accepting new participants, so it's only a matter of looking up a trial that interests you and that is taking place in your area, and then contacting the primary researcher for an evaluation. If you are qualified for the study, the doctors will have you sign some paperwork full of disclosures, then oversee your care in relation to the study. The study I participated in was being conducted by my neurologist, which was great because I got to see her more often and got double the care for the regular price, since I didn't have to pay for the times that I saw her for the study. Check the appendix for some links to websites that list current studies.

Chapter XIV

Keep Doing What You're Doing

Many of us have lots of questions when we get diagnosed, and we can't help but to think about where our lives will be in a year or two, or ten. The questions in our heads can fill us with unnecessary worry. "How long will I be able to work?" "What if I'm in school or want to go back to school to retrain for something more Parkinson's-friendly?" "Can I still travel, experience nightlife, and be involved in sports?" These questions are difficult for us to answer, because everyone is different and everyone progresses differently with the disease.

It's also important to note that everyone will be in a different place when it comes to letting their work know about their illness. Luckily, most Western countries have laws that protect people with illnesses and disabilities, but this doesn't stop all problems. At best, some of these laws and regulations help delay the inevitable.

Work

Some of us look at work as just a way to earn income and to support ourselves and our family. Others look at work as a part of their identity and cannot imagine themselves doing anything but what they're doing now. Unfortunately, with Parkinson's, the traditional ideas about work go out the window. Instead of looking at our next promotion, or maybe thinking about jumping into a new career that's more exciting or interesting, we're looking at how we can move forward in a less stressful job that we can do on our own time and in our own place.

This has been the case for many people I know with Parkinson's. Some have gone from being marketing executives at big companies to being copywriters working from home. Others went from being well-known academics, to taking early retirement and becoming volunteers at nonprofits. Yet, by the same token, there are many people I know who continue to work the same job even after diagnosis or with years into the disease.

Ultimately, the disease will catch up with you, so it's best to plan ahead regarding what you want to do when the time comes to leave your job. One question many people have is, should you tell your boss that you have Parkinson's after diagnosis? Will this help set the stage for accommodations and a transition out of the company eventually, or will it lead to discrimination and prejudice, causing an immediate layoff (illegal, by the way, but difficult to prove).

Will Revealing Your Diagnosis at Work Lead to Career Suicide?

When I was diagnosed with Parkinson's in 2011 at age 33, I was full-swing into my teaching career. That all changed once the symptoms became too much for an ambitious young academic to bear. I suddenly went from being outspoken and involved to being someone who barely had the stamina to make it through an 8am lecture. I thought my career was over. I decided I'd need to disclose my diagnosis since it was obvious that something was wrong. To my school's credit, they sought to accommodate me by switching me to teaching online courses. I knew my dream of becoming a full faculty member was likely over, but at least I could still teach and write.

While I was able to continue working in a more limited capacity, many of my friends in the Parkinson's community have not been so lucky. My support groups are filled with examples of people diagnosed in their 40s and 50s, and asked to retire or who mysteriously became the only victim of an unplanned layoff. This type of discrimination is illegal but proving it's extremely difficult and often not worth the stress to someone with serious health problems.

By 2015, I had sufficiently grieved the loss that came with being diagnosed with the Ballsy Palsy, and I thought it was time I tried to be more of my old self again. For me, this meant fighting back against the illness – staying fit and healthy, and beginning to advocate for others with Parkinson's. In order to be an advocate for people with Parkinson's – to raise awareness of the illness, support efforts for a cure, help others with the illness, and help develop empathy in those without the illness – I knew I'd need to go public with my diagnosis. I began writing online articles about Parkinson's and I began associating my name with the disease. I'm well aware that anything published on the internet is likely to be up for all time, so this bears the question: Am I sabotaging my own future by so publicly revealing my diagnosis and by being so public about it? Will future employers search my name online, find this book, and find out I have Parkinson's? Actually, I certainly hope so. Here's why.

I have Parkinson's and I can't hide it. What is the use of keeping my illness private if it's quite literally written on my face? Hiding it could make sense if I lived in a small town, on a farm, by myself, and wanted to be left alone. But I don't live on a farm. Instead, I live a somewhat public life through my writing, my teaching, my advocacy and political work, and on social media. If we meet in person, the elephant in the room, so to speak, is out of the way, and we can move forward immediately.

Future employers can see how hard I work on things I'm passionate about. Everyone seems to want to curate and control their online presence these days, and for good reason. Employers are known to look at social media to see what their applicants and employees are sharing publicly. Searching my name will return results about this book, my apps, my website, and the interviews I've given. I believe this would be an asset to an employer!

Instant recognition. Back when I was trying to hide my illness from the public, I had an experience that really affected me negatively and changed my thinking. In 2013, I decided to apply for the MBA program at the University of Washington. Not telling them about my illness, I was invited to their group interviews – essentially, I looked good on paper, and they wanted to know me in person. I hadn't started taking medications at that time, and after struggling with stiffness and slow movements, I was later rejected from the program because they said I seemed "bored and disinterested." I tried to explain my illness to the program directors and asked them to reconsider but they would not. The next year I applied again, making my illness clear in every essay and during the group interview. This time I was accepted and eventually was voted by my class as class representative, won a social entrepreneurship competition and was well respected by my peers and by the program officials. The bottom line: without sharing my illness, I never would have even gotten my foot through the door.

Living an authentic life. I'm very much into living an authentic life. I consider myself an honest and loyal person, someone who values fairness, and who wears his emotions on his sleeve. I'm not interested in hiding something like a major illness from the world. For better or for worse, Parkinson's and I are connected, likely for life. Everything I do in life will be viewed in light of the fact that I have Parkinson's. In many ways, this brings purpose to everything I do. For example, I have run for public office in the past, and if it seems appropriate, I may so again. The people who are my would-be constituents must know that having this illness, I don't take on obligations or projects willy-nilly. Instead, I ask myself "can I make a difference," and only commit if I know I can. If I run for public office again, it would be with the fervent desire to work with purpose, or else I'd see no point. The same is true for anything I do in my life.

I believe that revealing my illness to the world does more good than bad. While I'm worried that I might be underestimated by someone who doesn't understand Parkinson's, I'm not afraid to be labeled as someone with an illness – having Parkinson's has led me to help inspire thousands of people struggling with this disease, so I wear it as a badge of honor.

In the end, the right answer is different for everyone, but there are some things you can consider when deciding whether to tell your boss. If you have a good relationship with your boss, and you feel that they would be your advocate in trying to find accommodations for you, it may be worth telling them, especially if your symptoms are very noticeable. If your symptoms are not noticeable or you don't have a good relationship with your boss or you feel like your job might be on thin ice, it may be better not to share that information. Again, discrimination against illness and disability is illegal in most countries, but this doesn't stop employers from finding a reason to lay you off or have you fired – I have seen it done too many times.

In my situation, I taught students in a classroom at the college and university, and thanks to the advent of online learning and online courses that most higher education institutions have adopted, I was able to transition to teaching online the same classes that I taught on campus.

So what if now you can no longer work in the job you have had for the last 20 or 30 years, but you still need to make income? What can you do next? You can take a hint from my own story, and recognize that the Internet can be used as a tool to perform work from a distance. Most office jobs today can be done remotely from home. All you need is a newer computer, Skype, and know how to use software like word processors, spreadsheets, email and web browsers. The more you know about the options that are out there, the more you can use your knowledge to lobby your company to switch you to remote status. And even if your company doesn't want to do that for you, you can use your existing office skills from home working for other companies as a contractor. This allows you to work at your own pace on your own timetable, and when you are feeling well enough to do it. I have some remote work resources in the appendix to help get you started.

Now you may be asking, "what if I don't have an office job?" "What if I work out in the field in a job that requires physical strength and endurance?" Well, unfortunately with Parkinson's, working in a job that requires physical strength and endurance, or that may be physically stressful, will not be a long-term option for you. If you are someone who is young-onset, and in your 30s or 40s, your best option would be to transition to a job that is less physically strenuous and that can be done on your own timetable and schedule. One option is going back to school to retrain in a career that lends itself to remote work.

I know that for myself, I could no longer be on a schedule teaching classes and taking meetings like I used to. What if my class met on Mondays and Wednesdays at 8am and I wake up on Monday morning and I feel horrible. I'm essentially abandoning 120 students, since it's nearly impossible to find a substitute with an hour's notice. It's not fair to me, it's not fair to students, and it's not fair to the school. When I work from home, there is some amount of work I need to do each week, but the times that I can do that work are flexible. This means that if I have a rough night that leads to a rough morning, I can do the work I need to do in the afternoon or the next day when I'm feeling better and my meds are working.

Thanks to the gig economy, there are a whole new set of jobs available for PWPs that can be done whenever you're feeling up to it. If you want to do office work, the website Upwork (upwork.com) can help you find part-time, short-term jobs that you can do in your spare time. You can also deliver groceries with Instacart (instacart.com), walk dogs with Rover (rover.com), and even drive people around with Uber (uber.com). Just like Parkinson's isn't only an old person disease, these gig sites aren't just for young people. Anyone who needs a flexible schedule and can only work a certain number of hours can make money by becoming a freelancer on one of these platforms. When you're feeling up for it, you make yourself available on the app, and when you are having a rough day, you simply turn it off.

Remember, with Parkinson's, you have a new priority in your life: your health comes first. You will have no job if you can't keep yourself as healthy as possible. If what you're doing now for work is too much for you and it's unsustainable in the long-term, there are alternatives like retraining for a more Parkinson's-compatible career.

Keep Learning

Let's say that you have just taken early retirement from the job that you have been at for 30 years, or you're in your mid-30s or mid-40s and Parkinson's has become too much of a burden for you to work regular hours at your regular job. Or let's say that you're in your 60s or 70s, and feel like your mind is not active enough and you would like to do more to exercise your cognition. This is the perfect time to learn a new skill that can help you to improve your career prospects, or just to improve your life. Going back to school to retrain for a remote working environment, or simply learning a new language, can help you find new fulfillment in your life no matter what stage you are in.

If you decide that Parkinson's has become too much for you to hold a full-time regular office job, it may be time to retrain yourself in something that you can do from home and on your own time schedule. For me that was learning computer science. I enrolled in an online computer science program – the entire degree can be completed online, and once I graduate I can work remotely from home. I can offer my services on Upwork and work on my own time schedule and when I feel well enough, or I could work as an employee for a company that allows me to work from home. I could also use my skills to create my own software products. Finally, computer programming offers me the mental challenge I'm so in need of after leaving my in-person teaching career. The new skill you acquire may be different than mine since it should be interesting to you. Perhaps you've always been very good with words, so maybe you take a writing workshop to learn how to write articles for blogs or online magazines. I know several people that work from home writing articles for online publications.

Perhaps you are not interested in retraining in a new area, but you simply would like to keep your mind active. One of the best ways I know of to keep your mind active is to learn a new language. Learning a new language has been shown to help create new connections between neurons in your brain. Even into our later years of life, our brain remains moldable and neurons are still being created. You can learn a new language at home from your smart phone or computer using software like Duolingo, or you can go to language classes at community centers or junior colleges. This is also a great way to meet new people and feel like you are still a part of society. Learning a new language also has the obvious benefit of gaining the ability to communicate with an entirely new group of people and to experience different cultures. Imagine yourself learning Chinese, Hindi, or French, each of which is spoken natively by over a billion people around the world!

Another reason why lifelong learning is so important, especially for PWPs, is because it's important to have life goals, at any age. By definition, a goal is forward looking and indicates a positive outlook on life. Having goals gives us something to strive for, that why that keeps us going. By creating goals for ourselves, we are saying "I'm not done yet." This attitude also fosters optimism, which is something we definitely need when we are battling this illness.

Social Life

When we are young and inexperienced about the world, we tend to think that our work and our possessions are among the most important things in our lives. It's only later in life that we realize that this is not the case. Rather, the people around us are what make life matter. Having lunch with a friend you've had since childhood, or taking a road trip with family – these are the things that matter most because those relationships will be there long after you no longer work and after your possessions have become obsolete. This is why it's important to maintain strong social interactions as we get older. Although we may tend to want to hide away from the world, we must fight to do the opposite. After your top priority of caring for your health, your next highest obligation to yourself is nurturing your best relationships – those with your partner, family, and friends.

For PWPs, having people around us is the key to well-being. Whether you are an introvert or extrovert, being surrounded by people that we care about and who care about us is going to make us live healthier and longer lives. Having experiences with loved ones is often what keeps us going in the face of such a challenge. Sharing stories about the past, talking about the day-to-day, and thinking about the near future activities in which we will participate, will all make us feel that we are still a part of a tribe. Humans have evolved to be a part of tribes, and even in ancient times people who lived in tribes lived longer that those who were more nomadic. Our ancient ancestors stuck together to avoid the grittiness of the world. This is necessary for our survival today as well.

Besides the fact that connecting one-on-one with the people we care about most is important to keep us going, being around people who can help us get through life will be especially important as our own mobility decreases. Even if we have considered ourselves self-sufficient throughout our whole lives, Parkinson's has other plans for us. Having someone to help us out to make the occasional dinner, or to be available if an accident happens, is not only extremely

160

important but also vital. Not all of us are blessed to have friends and family nearby, but it's important to seek out this type of assistance, even professionally when possible. Some healthcare plans and most long-term care plans pay for in-home assistance, so it's worth looking into this if you need help with different aspects of your home life.

It's also important to do your part in keeping in step with society. It's easy to get into thinking that having Parkinson's will inevitably lead to you being estranged from the world, and you may feel like your symptoms are so bad that you think that you should stay away from people. This the wrong attitude! Getting sick is the wrong time to become a hermit. People who shut themselves in and shut other people out are less likely to live long, healthy lives. I definitely have those days I just want to stay home and watch TV when my tremor is bad or when my dyskinesias get out of hand. I feel a cringe when I can sense people watching me walk funny or sloppily eating a burrito, but I still do it. Let them think what they want to think. As Rosaline likes to remind me, "Who are these people to you? You don't know them, why do you care so much what they think?" She has also come up with some funny phrases to tell people who stare, like "Why don't you take a picture, it'll last longer!" Ironically, even being around people who stare when they see someone showing Parkinson's symptoms is important. Perhaps they have never known someone with Parkinson's. Now they see it first hand, which helps build awareness and even helps develop empathy. If people stare, let them stare. Maintaining your connection to the community is much more important than whether someone is being overly-curious about your dyskinesia. Seeing life happen around us brings us closer to our connection with humanity. In fact, I'll often go to a café when I'm not doing well, just to sit there and have a coffee around other people. This does wonders for the mind, the heart, and the soul.

Unfortunately, I've met people in the Parkinson's community who have decided they would rather shy away from social interactions. They order groceries and other necessities online and have them delivered. They don't keep in contact with friends or loved ones because they feel it has become too much of an effort, or because they don't want to burden others with their problems. They never go out and have just attached themselves to their televisions or computers. In these cases, they have no one to talk to when their symptoms worsen. They begin feeling awkward around other people, and this becomes a vicious cycle – the less they go out, the more awkward they feel, which makes them want to go out even less. Whenever I feel like I may be insulating myself from other people, I'll immediately go out and have a conversation with someone just for fun. I'll go to the café or the corner store and strike up a conversation with the cashier about the weather or just to ask how their day is going. That 30-second interaction is usually enough to reconnect me to the world and my role in it.

Not only should you actively work to avoid becoming a hermit, you should actually work to open yourself up to others as much as possible. As PWPs, we carry a lot of pain inside, and by opening ourselves up to others, we become vulnerable to them and they in turn will become vulnerable to us, helping to forge an even deeper connection. These are connections that will keep us going, these empathetic relationships that we end up relying on for our own well-being.

Some of the most enduring friendships I have formed over the last several years have been with other PWPs. We started with something in common that will never change: we all have Parkinson's. From there, we saw what other commonalities we had. With one older gentleman, we both found joy in playing games like pool and pinball. We would meet together in bars in downtown Seattle to play pool, we would talk about Parkinson's, but also about life, politics, and a whole lot more. We were both open to discussing our thoughts about the illness and this helped foster connectedness. Another friend of mine happened to work in startups. We actually knew a lot of the same people in the startup community, and we were able to help each other out professionally, but we could also just get together to have dinner. He actually turned out to be interested in politics as well, so I introduced him to some of my political friends. These relationships would not have been possible without having had an open mindset along with a willingness to seek connections with the broader world.

Accommodations

Most countries have some sort of disability act that ensures that people with disabilities have access to services, facilities, etc. In the United States, the Americans with Disabilities Act exists to do just that for Americans. These laws not only assure that business' doors are of a certain weight to make them easy for anybody to open, but also to ensure that if you become disabled, your employer or your school must attempt to make reasonable accommodations for your disability. This is tricky with Parkinson's, because the degree of disability and the related accommodations are likely to be different for each person. For example, a company accommodating a visually impaired employee may have a standard set of accommodations that they have likely used with other visually impaired employees. On the other hand, there is so much variation with Parkinson's, that it's typically up to the PWP to know what type of accommodations are necessary. Even if you know what accommodations work well for you, you may face resistance from your accommodations coordinator. After all, how do you accommodate someone who cannot use their hands due to tremors, thinks a little bit more slowly, cannot sit for longer than a couple of hours at a time, and requires afternoon naps? This is not as easy to accommodate. Not to mention that some symptoms are more severe in some people than in others, that symptoms change intensity from day to day, and that these symptoms get worse over time.

The most important thing to remember when you are in need of accommodations is to actually request those accommodations. If you are at the point at which you need accommodations, and it would be impossible to do your job or go to school without them, then you should request accommodations as soon as possible. Many people wait until their symptoms start showing to let their work know about the disease, or about the need for accommodations. That's fine, but once you let them know, they are on notice that you are someone with special needs. At larger companies, you would likely work with a coordinator in HR to work out accommodations. In smaller companies, you may be dealing directly with your boss. In schools, entire departments exist ready to help you succeed by accommodating your needs.

While we are discussing accommodations, it's also useful to discuss what happens when your requested accommodations are not met, or if there is a case of discrimination. If you believe that your rights have been violated, by discrimination or in some other form, and you cannot resolve the issue by discussing it with your organization, you may want to discuss your case with an attorney. Your doctor may have a recommendation for an attorney, or you could reach out to your support group or support group leader for recommendations. Keep in mind, it's the law (certainly in the United States, but also in many other western countries) for employers and other institutions to make an attempt to make reasonable accommodations for you. This may mean buying a special chair and pointing device for your computer, but it may not mean giving you free reign to come in and leave whenever you want. One may be reasonable and one may not be reasonable according to your employer.

A couple of PWPs I know have been laid off or fired shortly after asking for accommodations. This is, of course, illegal, and can be brought to an attorney for legal remedy. Some employers may use the fact that they are at-will employers as a defense. In theory, this means that they are allowed to hire and fire employees at-will, for any reason. However, it is illegal to fire someone, even in an at-will situation, because of a disability. One person I know was fired shortly after she disclosed her disability, even though she had worked there for 10 years. She decided to not bring a case against the company, but could have. For many people, however, seeking legal action may not be worth the stress and cost.

Ultimately, we should recognize that Parkinson's limits us in some ways. It may be possible that we can't do the same job we used to do, even with accommodations. It's at this point we need to decide what we want to do next in our lives. If you were younger when you were first diagnosed, like I was, you may want to consider doing different work in your field, but that takes your limitations into account. Or, you may be like many people I have met and decide to switch careers altogether.

Just one more note about schools and institutions of higher learning; all schools in the United States are subject to laws regarding the Americans with Disabilities Act, but the laws are more significant for schools receiving federal aid. In these cases, you may file an ADA complaint with the

Department of Justice, and they will investigate the case for you. Public schools are aware that being found guilty of discriminating against a student (or faculty member) could mean losing their federal funding and/or accreditation.

Disability

There may come a time in your Parkinson's voyage in which you say, "enough is enough" when it comes to work (but never about life!). You have tried your best, you asked for accommodations, you changed your work schedule, and you are still having difficulties and are unable to do the job the way it should be done or not to your satisfaction. This is the point when you may consider retiring and filing for disability. Most countries offer disability benefits for those who cannot continue working. In the United States, this usually comes from Social Security or a pension fund.

The process for filing for disability is not fun. You will be asked to have a doctor's recommendation for disability, and you will need to fill out lots of forms. The people who decide on disability benefits are ready to say "no" as soon as they receive your application, mainly to prevent ineligible applicants from abusing the system. This is why it's recommended you speak to an attorney before beginning the process. In the United States, there are attorneys who specialize in disability, and who do not recover a fee until after the applicant has been approved, and even then, there is a limit on how much they can charge. Be careful with attorneys who want to charge upfront fees or will make you pay regardless of whether you get approved or not.

Your attorney will guide you through the process and have you go see your doctor for a recommendation. The doctor will examine you and decide whether you're eligible for disability or not. When you're at your doctor's appointment, you should tell them about how you feel during the good times as well as the bad times. Don't gloss over the bad times, since that is the part that makes you eligible for disability. Make sure you tell your doctor exactly what is preventing you from working and why you should be granted disability. Be truthful, and be sure your doctor records your responses accurately.

Your attorney will help you file the paperwork along with your doctor's notes. Understand that the process can take a long time. Sometimes it may take up to six months before you even hear back from Social Security. It's actually quite common for applicants to be rejected on the first attempt at filing for disability. In this case, the attorney can help you file an appeal for reconsideration. If you are indeed disabled and cannot work, disability is typically granted no later than on the first appeal.

Once you are approved, you will receive a monthly stipend, which is some percentage of your income before becoming disabled, and access to the socialized healthcare system your country has to offer. You may also be eligible for reduced-cost housing, disability placards for your vehicle, and reduced-cost or free public transport. In addition, if you have federally subsidized student loans, those may be forgiven. You are typically allowed to earn a certain amount of income per month, but this varies by jurisdiction so check with your local laws. I have one friend who is disabled and delivers groceries once a week through Instacart, just to have a little extra spending money and to get out of the house for a couple of hours.

Chapter XV

Thriving

While in the past I have felt like I was simply surviving while the disease overtook my body, today I feel that I'm truly thriving. Although Seattle was a wonderful city to live in, I have moved once again, this time to Amsterdam, for a brand-new adventure with Rosaline. I feel healthier, more fit, and more hopeful for the future than I have in nearly a decade of this Parkinson's adventure. Going from deep depression to thriving didn't happen accidentally; it was a long process, and it took a lot of work. We only live once, and I was not going to spend most of it sulking and suffering.

I discussed earlier about how I discovered the meaning of life. The secret, the one that everybody wishes they knew, is simple.

The meaning of life is to enjoy life.

That's it. It's that simple. Of course, enjoying life has a different meaning for everyone, but I believe everyone is capable of achieving joy. For me, the biggest aspect of enjoying life means spending time with my family and friends, especially my wife, and having new adventures. I'm not suggesting leading a hedonistic life with only fun and parties. Other things that bring me immense joy are teaching students, writing, helping people in the community, and having optimism about the future. Inherent in the idea of enjoying life is to find happiness in the current moment – not living in the past, but also not planning so far ahead in the future. Happiness is a choice you have to make for yourself.

I have chosen happiness. I understand that Parkinson's is a part of me – I do not have it and it does not have me. Parkinson's is simply an aspect of my life that I must contend with, but when my obituary is written, "Nick was afflicted with Parkinson's" should be the last line of that obituary, not the first. The first line will read something like, "Author, traveler, dreamer, Nick was all these things."

Be who you were always meant to be – don't let Parkinson's stop you from that. Say it, believe it, live it, and it will be so. Did I waste nearly a decade of my life feeling sorry for myself? Yes, but I have no time for the past. Might I end up in a wheelchair in 10 or 20 years? Maybe, but I'm traveling to Paris and Milan soon so I have no time to worry about what might happen in the distant future.

If you want to live this way as well, there are a few things you need to do.

Stay Positive

One of the biggest determining factors for how your body reacts to Parkinson's is your mood. Being grumpy and having a bad mood plays into the severity of symptoms. This is why it's very important to stay positive. If your mood is up and you are thinking positive thoughts, your body will follow. Many times, staying positive is easier said than done.

Sometimes it may be easy to get down, like when you meet someone in advanced stages at a support group meeting. It's hard not to think of yourself being in that person's condition sometime down the line. But this is the wrong way to look at the situation. You have this moment right now to live your life. Go out there and live it. When we live in the now and practice mindfulness – stopping to smell the roses, as they say – it's much easier to stay positive.

Staying positive also has another benefit: the people around you will see your positivity and will respond with positivity. Some people may also recognize your positive attitude in light of your struggles and see you as an inspiration. We tend to think that once we are stricken with some serious condition our usefulness has disappeared, but nothing could be further from the truth. The joy you bring to the world when you are sick is so powerful. Be thankful for the life you have now, as well as for the people you have around you. You will live a longer, better life in every respect.

Be Grateful

In life, it's often too easy to take the great things in our lives for granted. We often expect our loved ones to be there when we need them, just as reliably as the sun rises each day. It's also easy to take for granted the days that you're feeling well, especially if you had been having some bad days. In both of these situations, and in life in general, it pays to be grateful. Be grateful for the health that you have now instead of crying over the life you used to have. Be grateful that your eyes can open and that your lungs can breathe, and that you have warm blood coursing through your veins. Gratitude is something we don't think about enough, but when we show gratitude to the world, the world takes notice.

A few years after being diagnosed, my symptoms became very pronounced and I became unable to do some basic things for myself. Up until this point, I had always been independent and too proud (read: stubborn) to ask for help. I decided I'd swallow my pride and ignore my ego, and ask for help from those around me. At the supermarket, I began asking for help getting items off the top shelf or even just opening up the plastic produce bag. Anytime someone would help me, I'd be sure they knew I was grateful. Beyond just saying "thanks," which would most often garner a sincere "you're welcome," I'd say "thank you so much. I really appreciate it." Just saying these extra words, words people don't seem to use enough these days, I'd get responses like "oh, you're so welcome. It's my pleasure." The interaction went from being a stranger helping a disabled person to being more about two humans exercising their humanity.

It's easy to get caught up in our busy and messy lives, and it just seems easier to coast and take the great things around us for granted. Our loved ones are likely the ones who hear of our gratitude the least, but should hear about it the most. Rosaline and I have had this conversation. She helps me with something and I say thank you, and she says "well, we're married, and it's part of my job." Then I tell her that I really appreciate her and everything she does and for me. Our loved ones know us, and they understand when we are grateful for their help, but it's nice to hear that verbal acknowledgement sometimes. Gratitude can also be unspoken, like making breakfast in bed on a Sunday or buying a dozen roses every once in a while.

So as we can see, there are two types of gratitude. The internal gratitude, in which you thank your body and yourself for being alive, even though life may not be all roses, and then there is the external gratitude, in which we show others how much we appreciate them and their love and attention. Both are important and both are best when exercised daily.

Know Yourself

Keeping high spirits is very difficult when you wake up in the morning and you can't move well. It's important to know what your weaknesses are, physically, emotionally, cognitively, etc. Understand when your best times and worst times happen. If you can't get out of bed in the morning, and each morning feels like the world is coming to an end, but then you feel better in the afternoon, knowing that is very important for how you plan your day and how you make decisions.

Of course, it's also difficult to know yourself and to also act on that knowledge. We're only human, and we all make mistakes. Sometimes we ignore what we know in order to feel a certain way in the short term, while putting ourselves in jeopardy in the longer term. Just because we have self-knowledge it doesn't mean we use it. At times when I feel upset with the world, I'll have moments where I no longer want to interact with others, or I don't want to show any gratitude for being alive. It's important to catch ourselves in those moments and spend the time we need in order to reset our mindset and return to our baseline. It's important to keep track of when these episodes happen so we can recognize the patterns and anticipate them in the future. Keeping a journal with your daily thoughts can help with this, and so can keeping track of your mood at different times of the day and over time.

Another important aspect of having good mind-body health is allowing yourself to have an illness. I know I'm not the same person I was 10 or 20 years ago. I wouldn't be the same person even if I didn't have Parkinson's. I'm a different person with different ideals, different experiences, and different goals. Just as I have had to accept the fact that I'm getting older and that opportunities are no longer available to me because of age, I have to allow the same for the disease. There are simply things I cannot do. Although I love to travel, I'll never make it on a trip around the world in 80 days. Although I love playing pinball, I'll never be number one or maybe even top thousand in the world. Although I love starting businesses, my body doesn't allow me to run a start-up with investors breathing down my neck. As someone with a chronic illness, I have to give myself permission to be okay with my limitations. I need to be okay with the fact that I can't do those things, and that this doesn't mean that my life is over. I can still travel at a slower pace. I can still play pinball and have good time, I can still start small businesses that I run more as a hobby. I can still do a lot, but it's important to set the right expectations.

Accepting that you have an illness that limits you in some ways is different than giving up on yourself and on your dreams. Instead, it's coming to terms with this fact and acting accordingly to avoid disappointment. You have likely gone through the five stage of grief, and you now realize that you need to readjust your goals in life to meet this new reality. However, don't use this as an excuse to stop reaching for your goals and achieving your dreams. Coming to terms just means you need to take a different route and make sure you take care of yourself as well. Changing your mindset from someone who can't do something to someone who needs to find a different way to do something is a very powerful and positive attitude change to make. It's like making the distinction between someone who says "I'm depressed," to someone who says "I'm a person experiencing feelings of depression." Parkinson's is not you, and you are not Parkinson's. Parkinson's is something that accompanies you. You are still yourself. You can still be ambitious, productive, and successful with Parkinson's, you just have to reframe how you see things.

I've already said this but it's worth repeating: we are all just human. I know that exercise will help slow the progression of Parkinson's, but some days or some weeks I'm just not feeling it and I don't do any exercise. I know that I have my ups and downs and that some days I'll feel better than others, but I can still feel like it's the end of the world when I'm having a particularly down day. It's okay. We need to allow ourselves these indiscretions and forgive ourselves. We are not perfect, and that's okay.

Sometimes I feel pretty useless when my drugs are not working. I lay in bed and have difficulty moving. My hands shake and my muscles feel stiff. Eventually when my medications come on, I'll want to be unproductive and just lay down instead of using that on-time to do work. This is something that I should allow myself to do: being on and knowing I can be productive but choosing instead to rest comfortably. Much of what I do is more about self-preservation and less about being as productive as I can be. Maybe I'm saving my energy for later, or maybe I just want to rest my body while I'm "on." You may be unproductive when it comes to work or chores, but you are being productive for your illness.

In my case, knowing myself means understanding that I'm not a morning person. I have a policy of never making important decisions for at least three hours after waking up in the morning. Sometimes I wake up especially tired or off because I overslept or because I missed my evening dose of medication. But once I get up and get going, have breakfast, and take my medications, I start to feel much better. My medicated body starts thinking with a positive lens, and only then do I trust myself with making important decisions.

I also never make appointments for any time before noon, since I know that my body needs a few hours to get going. Keep track of your mood in a diary or using the Parkinson's LifeKit app to find out when your ideal time of day is, and adjust your lifestyle accordingly.

Part of knowing your limitations includes choosing in which activities to be involved. If you know that taking a 6-mile hike will leave you completely exhausted for three days, or that taking a night class twice a week leaves you unable to wake up early the next morning, then don't do those things. It's important to learn about your body's ups and downs and its triggers, so you can make better decisions.

Minimize Stress

Just as exercise is the one thing scientifically known to slow the progression of Parkinson's, the one thing that is known to accelerate the decline is stress. Stress is a killer for Parkinson's disease, perhaps not literally, but it definitely is very harmful to our bodies and minds. Doctors are very adamant about stress-avoidance. My neurologist says that I should try to eliminate as much stress as possible in my life. That's easy for her to say! Parkinson's is stressful, and it's often accompanied with depression and disappointment; it's all too easy to focus on all of the things Parkinson's has taken from us. But knowing that the stress exists, it's important to minimize the stress in your life as much as possible. If you are nearing retirement age, it may be worthwhile to consider early retirement. If you were diagnosed earlier in life like I was, retirement is often not a realistic option, but it's still possible to make choices that eliminate unnecessary stressors from your life.

What is stress anyways? Stress happens when there is a gap between our responsibilities and our capabilities. With this definition, it's easy to see why stress manifests itself in PWPs; our responsibilities have not changed – we still need to work, take the kids to school, feed ourselves, etc. – but our capabilities to do these things have decreased. The gap between what we need to do and what we can do has just gotten bigger.

Stress comes in two main flavors – good stress and bad stress. Good stress is when we challenge ourselves and we are enjoying life. An example is taking a family trip – Parkinson's has made the travel a lot more difficult, but you are excited and spending time with loved ones. Good stress puts pressure on our bodies, but we are also feeling the dopamine and endorphins flowing through our bloodstreams. Another example of good stress is working out – our bodies are again under pressure, but our blood is flowing and the workout leaves us feeling refreshed and healthier. One "good stress" activity I enjoy is going to support groups, especially the active ones where we go for a walk or hike and then visit a bar or a cafe for some snacks and discussion. Having social interactions with people facing the same challenges as you actually helps relieve bad stress.

Bad stress happens when we are challenged in a situation that's imperative to our lives and lifestyle – work is becoming too difficult, relationships are becoming strained, feeding and bathing yourself has become problematic. These situations put pressure on our bodies but they are accompanied by anger and other negative emotions. Other bad stressors to lookout for include having a bad boss, or having to hide your disease at work. These bad stressors can lead to a faster decline. We don't want that!

Don't Worry

Worry is anxiety about a future that has not happened yet. If the future has not happened, you have no control over it, so why worry? You may say, "I don't know how my disease will progress." While this is true, there is no telling how your disease will or will not progress – you have no control over the future. You only control the moment now. If you feel that your disease may progress badly, do something about it today. Every day is a new day to make a difference in your life. Exercising, choosing a healthy lunch option, researching the disease – those things happen in the now, not in the future. Do what you can today, and don't worry about a future that may not even come.

In psychology, there is the concept of a self-fulfilling prophecy. This means that if you believe hard enough that something will happen, then it ends up happening. If you believe that you are destined to crumble at a young age from Parkinson's, then you will subconsciously do everything in your power to make that real. You won't exercise, you won't worry about what you're eating, you won't pay attention to your mind or body. And then your prediction comes true. A self-fulfilling prophecy. If you stay positive and don't worry, saying to yourself that you will fight and make it through this, your mind will work to make it so. Keep worry out, and replace it with the beauty of the now.

Don't Regret

Just like worry is anxiety about a future that hasn't happened yet, regret is dwelling on things that have happened in the past. "I should have done this, I should have done that." What is the use of thinking about the past if you can't change it? We only have the now, today. The past is irrelevant. You can't change it, so there is no use dwelling on it. Take the past as prologue; the past is the little bit at the beginning of the story that sets up the rest of your life. Think about what lessons the past has taught you, and how those lessons can help guide you in the future. We've all made mistakes, but sometimes we don't learn from those mistakes, so we are bound to repeat them. The past is passed.

For a long time, I regretted not finishing that Masters of Business Administration. I had become so attached to the idea of completing the degree, that leaving the program completely destroyed me. I was depressed for a year after that, and shut myself off from everything connected to it, including my former classmates. It was the first time in my life I felt I had really failed at something. The entire experience was a blow to my character and ego. But looking back on it today, I don't regret having gone to the program, and I don't regret leaving when I left. I didn't leave because I had just given up, although having Parkinson's is good enough reason to give up on big undertakings sometimes. I left because my body failed me. This is nothing to be ashamed of. I tried my best, I made an impact while I was there, and I left when my body said "enough is enough." I'm glad to have had that experience; it taught me a lot about myself and about life.

Redefine Productivity

As a PWP, you are probably familiar with the unfinished to-do list. "Today I'm going to write a few e-mails, do the dishes, organize the holiday decorations, and take a walk through the garden." The afternoon flies by and suddenly it's bedtime. Except we have completed only half of the items on the list. How can we get anything done?

Rather than feel like life is moving too fast, or that we are moving too slowly and getting nothing done, it's a better idea to redefine what productivity means for a PWP.

Whether you're still working full time or just doing chores around the house, you have one boss that matters more than any other: your body. Your body's well-being is your number one priority, and it will dictate how much you can get done. Whether you subscribe to the idea of spoon theory (in which you imagine having a given number of spoons per day, and each activity costs you spoons until you have none left, and going beyond that limit means borrowing from tomorrow's spoons) or any other way of measuring your body's limits, learn your own limitations and adhere to them.

Spread It Out

When building your to-do list, make a list of things to do over a certain period of time like a week, not just for one day. This will take some planning, but it ensures that you won't feel bad about not getting things done when you are not feeling well. It also gives you a chance to fit in some extra activities on a day you are feeling especially well. For example, my list contains "go to the market" twice a week. If I'm not feeling well on Tuesday, I can always go on Wednesday or Thursday. I plan ahead by keeping a few frozen entrees in the freezer for those days I should have shopped but wasn't feeling up for it. I also always keep at least a week's worth of dry goods and canned veggies on hand so I can always whip up an easy pasta dish without having to go out. I've also embraced grocery and restaurant home delivery services.

Change Expectations

Consider changing your expectations of yourself, especially if you are constantly behind on your to-do list. You don't have the same energy or stamina you had before your diagnosis, so plan accordingly. Give yourself permission to do less. Whenever I'm about to add an item to my to-do list, I ask myself "do I really need to do this?" Sometimes I just want to stay busy, but it's worth spending more time on one or two things than spreading myself thin doing too much. It's been very useful for me to eliminate distractions and busy work to focus on doing just a couple of things well. We're not as independent as we used to be, and that can be the most difficult pill to swallow for most of us. Don't be embarrassed or afraid to ask for help. You with something at home, to asking a stranger to grab an item off of the shelf at the supermarket, people are willing to help.

Keep Your Thoughts Organized

My to-do list used to contain everything that needed to get done around the house and every errand I needed to run, not to mention everything I needed to do for work. Just opening that list overwhelmed me. I solved this by breaking up the tasks into separate categories so I could focus on whatever I felt like doing at that moment. I also removed useless filler activities like "think about what type of bike to buy" or "go to the cafe for a macchiato" (I'm not kidding). I realized I needed a journal to keep my thoughts organized and to make notes about everyday life. Not all of your thoughts or ideas belong on your to-do list. This has helped me immensely with focus, helping me concentrate on what is really important.

Listen to Your Body

Understand that listening to your body is being productive. Your number one item on your to-do list should be "manage my health." That means that if your body asks for sleep, you are being productive by sleeping. If you absolutely must decide between washing dishes or going for a walk, choose the walk. It can be disappointing to have two or three things planned for your day and only end up doing one. This is our life now — embrace the change. Now I know that if I have something planned for the evening, I'll take it easy during the day. Listening to my body has really improved my quality of life and has made me cherish the things I do accomplish.

Ultimately, you will want to slow down in your everyday life. There are a lot of things to do in life — work, play, spend time with family and friends — but like it or not we have limitations we need to consider. By re-framing how we look at the idea of productivity and re-prioritizing what's important, we can make the changes needed to lead a fuller and happier life.

Don't Give Up on Yourself or Your Dreams

You may have heard the phrase the young people are saying these days, YOLO. It means, You Only Live Once. Although you have always known this, its meaning becomes more important as we think about living with a chronic illness. If we only have one life to live, are we choosing to live it? Are we going to allow Parkinson's to make us sit on the sofa and watch TV all day for the rest of our lives? Is that the life you always told yourself you would live? Sure, when we were children we would all be astronauts and race car drivers, but as we got older our dreams became more focused and our interests and desires more refined.

Think about who you were before you were diagnosed with Parkinson's. That year before your diagnosis – was there something you dreamt of doing or becoming? Were you on track to accomplish some big goal, professionally or personally? Is there any way that you can recapture that feeling and apply it to an activity you can do today? Have you ever said that you wanted to run your own business? You can still do that by selling on eBay or Etsy. You can do as little or as much as you would like, and do it on your own schedule. If you ever told yourself that you would have a beautiful garden, then why not do it? Even if you live in an apartment, you can find community gardens in your city where you can participate. People go out and work on the gardens together and share in the fruits of the labor. You can contribute as much or as little as you want. The point is, if you have the will to move forward with your dreams, there is a way to make those dreams a reality.

I'll take it a step further. When I was younger, I knew I wanted to change the world for the better. Then Parkinson's struck. And while I sometimes spend half the day in bed because my body is tired, I simply see those times as the necessary price to pay for trying to live my life to its full potential. When my body cooperates, I make apps that PWPs around the world are using to make their lives better. I wrote this book, which will hopefully improve the lives of PWPs and their loved ones around the world. I write on my personal blog at http://nickpernisco.com, and thousands of people have read my writings. I stand up and speak out for what I believe is right, getting involved with issues related to homelessness, poverty, health, and equality. The work I do is all done on my computer, which can easily be used in bed on a bad day, or at a café on a good day. On the days that I can't type, I use a dictation program called Dragon that has learned my speech patterns and allows me to dictate into my computer. It even understands when I slur words!

The point of all of this is that you should not give up on yourself or your dreams. Do not give up on who you were before Parkinson's – you are still the same person! Maybe you won't be an astronaut, and maybe your business won't become a Fortune 500 company, but don't be afraid to bring out the you that is still dying to get out. Today it's easier than ever to stay involved and make things happen for yourself thanks to technology. Don't let the world tell you that you are someone else or that you can't do something. You can still accomplish anything you put your mind to, and the planet still needs what you have to offer.

Finding the Courage to Move Forward

Ever since I was very young, I have looked towards the future. This makes perfect sense, having grown up in an era of rapidly changing technology and having been a fan of everything sci-fi related. I'd watch movies that would take place sometime in the future, excited about the great new things the future would bring. Any time some new gadget was announced, I'd anxiously await the release date. I couldn't wait to grow up, because the future – my future – looked amazing.

But as I got older, a shift began to occur. My sights were set, not 20 years in the future, but 10 years, then five years, until life became about living and surviving the present moment. Then suddenly, the shift in my perspective continued – I began thinking more and more about the past. I'd think about regrets over missed opportunities and alternate lives that could have been lived. I could point to several specific moments in my life in which a decision I made altered my path. I'd look back at how fickle I was with life, and how things could have been different if I had followed one specific path over another. I suppose we all have those thoughts from time to time as we get older.

The place most people don't live in, however, is the present. The here and now is really all we have. As the author Sam Harris said, "The past is a memory – It's a thought arising in the present. The future is merely anticipated – It's another thought arising now." This is something that took me a long time to understand and put into practice. The idea of living in the present moment is important for all of us, but it's especially important for someone living with a chronic illness like Parkinson's.

When I learned that Parkinson's would be my companion, likely for the long haul, something strange happened. My thoughts about my past and future changed. Now instead of the past being filled with regret and remorse, I realized that my past wasn't filled with mistakes, but instead with actions that provided me with important lessons. Perhaps I was being a bit nostalgic – after all, it's easy to think fondly of the past when you know your toughest days lie ahead. And then instead of being optimistic about the future, I began thinking about how horrible my body would be battered by this illness. I dreaded what the future would bring, for me and for my family.

I had become depressed and anxious, and with my mental state in disarray, my body followed. Everything became more difficult to do. It wasn't until I chose – and yes, you must choose – to live in the present that things began to change. What was the point of being depressed over lost youth and innocence? I had a good childhood, did good things in college, and had a fantastic career helping others. And why have anxiety over the future? I don't know if there will be a cure for Parkinson's in my lifetime. Worrying about how my body would change in the future was beginning to ruin my present.

A common refrain in the Parkinson's community is that a cure for Parkinson's is just around the corner, just a few years away. I constantly tell people that I think a cure for Parkinson's is about five to ten years away. I'd like to think this is true, but I've been saying this for about ten years now, and I don't think we are much closer to a cure than when I was first diagnosed. While the treatment of symptoms has improved – with advances in carbidopa-levodopa delivery as well as in Deep Brain Stimulation – a cure is still not on the horizon.

I read a lot about Parkinson's – a lot. I'm subscribed to multiple online news feeds that deliver the latest headlines, with a variety of scientific journals on my list along with several publications written for the general public. What I have found, which can offer hope but is also a source of frustration, is that most of the supposedly huge breakthroughs in Parkinson's research have all occurred using animal models. This means that potential cures are working on rats in a lab, but they have not been tested on humans. The reason this matters is because in almost all cases in Parkinson's research, animal brain models don't translate to humans. This makes sense. Our brains are much more complex than those of rats or even monkeys. I've learned to temper expectations and only get excited when I read that some new treatment has made it to Phase 2 clinical trials on humans (the treatment is deemed safe for humans and now they're testing for efficacy). A potential cure that reaches Phase 3 would be a real reason to celebrate!

The good news is that there is a lot of money and intellectual power behind the search for a cure for

Parkinson's. There are constantly new studies and clinical trials opening and in search of participants, and the steady stream of articles from my Parkinson's news feeds is also a source of hope. One important aspect of Parkinson's research that is worth noting is that finding a cure for other brain diseases could lead to new discoveries for Parkinson's as well. Many neurologists feel that diseases like Alzheimer's, MS, and ALS are somehow related with Parkinson's. Funding and research for other brain diseases will help the broader neurological community discover new treatments.

While I'm filled with optimism that a cure (or at least a so-called disease-modifying drug) can be developed in my lifetime, I'm also weary and a bit skeptical that our current health system and public policy will allow this to happen. It seems to me that pharmaceutical companies want to develop drugs that will be used by patients over a long period of time. There are few if any incentives for these companies to discover outright cures that rid people of the disease and then no longer need the product. It may sound cynical, but I have read news stories over many years that confirm that this is what happens inside of "big pharma." And while in the past various governments have pledged to support brain research, they underfund the research and render the work useless. Pardon me for using a cliché, but curing brain diseases like Parkinson's is a moon shot, and it needs the funding to go along with it.

As I mentioned already, while an outright cure may not be feasible due to the current health system and public policy in the United States, I feel more optimistic about the development of disease-modifying drugs that can slow, stop, or reverse Parkinson's. Many of these are in the works, and while these are not the holy grail cure most would hope for, I wouldn't at all mind taking a drug my entire life to keep Parkinson's at bay rather than continuing to just mask the symptoms while my body continues to worsen underneath. One such treatment is being developed in my recent home of Seattle at the University of Washington by a startup called M3 Biotechnology. I've spoken with the founder and CEO, Leen Kawas, and her work seems very promising.

For now, I take disease-masking drugs. Carbidopa-levodopa, Ropinerol, Rytary, and Amantadine all help hide Parkinson's from the world and help me continue to work, but none of them stop the progression. Underneath, my brain is still failing to produce the correct amount of dopamine my body needs, and it will only get worse. I'm glad these therapies exist, since I would not be able to even function without them. I would have long ago given up on life and would have just sat in a wheelchair waiting for it to be over. And while I have my struggles, I'm glad that I can still enjoy life with a newfound appreciation of what it has to offer.

So what does all this talk about no cure have to do with moving forward and living a good life? With the thought that my body could fail me at any time, and with no cure in the short-term, all I can do is stop worrying and start enjoying life. Whenever I feel sad or angry about the cards I have been dealt in life, I think about how lucky I was to not have been born somewhere in the world where I could have already died from poverty, hunger, or disease. I have a certain privilege that others don't, and I should not take that for granted and be upset about my own health problems, which seem insignificant by comparison. Keeping this idea top-of-mind helps keep me grounded in life, and also pushes me to help those who are less fortunate than I have been.

Plan for The Unexpected

Since Parkinson's is so unpredictable, and knowing that one day I may become completely disabled – it could be in five years or in 25 years – there are things that I have done to prepare for that day. The first step is setting up a living trust and putting all of our property in there. This ensures that Rosaline can do what she needs to do with our property if I'm not there. She also has power of attorney over me, so she can legally act for me in any situation if I'm unable. We handle our own financial planning, so we invest in low-risk mutual funds to have a degree of certainty about our finances no matter what the future brings. We have indicated our advanced directives, so she knows what I'd like to happen to me should I fall ill in a hospital. She even has all of my passwords in case she needs to access any of my online accounts. Parkinson's is unpredictable enough, having some certainty over legal and financial affairs can help take away a bit of the stress about what the future holds.

Now that this planning is done, I can forget about it. I have peace of mind that everything is in order, and I can focus on living my best life today.

Become an Advocate

There will come a time in your illness when you feel you have a handle on the Ballsy Palsy. You will have fewer bad days, or at least you will know how to handle the bad days when they show up. You will have gone through the Five Stages of Grief, and have come out the other side as a stronger, more determined person. You have not allowed Parkinson's to control you; you are a Parkinson's Warrior. So what's your next move, champ?

This is the time to become an advocate. Advocates write blog posts, shoot videos for YouTube, speak at gatherings large and small, and most of all they connect with other PWPs, all for the purpose of raising awareness, promoting understanding, and helping to find a cure. The internet makes this easy to do. While you can put your story out there for others to learn from, I've gotten the most satisfaction from interacting with individuals on a personal basis. In my nearly 10 years with the disease, I've seen almost everything Parkinson's can do to someone, and I have learned to live with it and thrive. This is why I enjoy connecting with people who have just been diagnosed. These newly-diagnosed PWPs are scared, anxious, depressed, are having family problems, etc. They have an endless number of questions about Parkinson's. They need reassurance, information, and a little inspiration. I can't fully express the joy it brings me to be able to be a new PWP's first contact and help them through the times I know were most difficult for me.

I see advocacy as a responsibility, as well as a natural next step after you have stabilized your own mind and body. The months after diagnosis is when PWPs feel the most alone and when they're likely to have the biggest rush of emotions. Having someone who has been through it all and who is willing to listen to them can help the PWP cope more easily at that moment. Become an advocate for the community, and be a mentor for a PWP who could use some guidance.

Don't Give Up

Hopefully, this book has given you a good overview of Parkinson's disease, and that my story has inspired you to continue on and keep fighting. This is the fight of your life, but it doesn't have to be all bad. I'm the prime example of how it's possible to live a good life with this disease. The choice of how to live with Parkinson's is yours. You can let it control you, or you can control it. There are times I've felt like giving up, but I kept pushing myself. Whether it was to prove something to the world, or to prove to myself that I was still worthy of being human and being alive, I worked around the limitations of Parkinson's, and continue to do so every single day of my life.

It's often said that people regret the things that they don't do in life, rather than the things they do. This has certainly been the case in my experience. When I was diagnosed with Parkinson's, my life was focused on accumulating things – a house, a car, the latest smartphone. But after my struggles, I realize that what I want most is experiences. Now I'm focused on having all types of experiences. I have started two software companies and a film production company. I have been on the radio and on television. I have written and published two books. I learned math late in life after I had failed at it so many times in my earlier years. I went to business school and started a non-profit. I have run for office and sat on committees, councils, and boards. I moved away from my hometown to another state, then several years later moved away across the world. I became an internationally ranked pinball player. And I did all these things after being diagnosed with Parkinson's disease. If I can do this, I feel I can do anything I put my mind to, and I believe you can as well.

Don't ever give up on yourself. Parkinson's is not you. Parkinson's is something that you carry with you, but doesn't have to define who you are. Live your life to the fullest and don't regret anything.

You only have one life to live, so go out and live it. YOLO!

Appendix A: Resources

Parkinson's Organizations

American Parkinson Disease Association
http://www.apdaparkinson.org/

Austrian Parkinson's Disease Society
http://www.parkinson.at/

Dallas Area Parkinsonism Society
http://www.daps.us/

Davis Phinney Foundation
http://www.davisphinneyfoundation.org/

European Parkinson's Disease Association
http://www.epda.eu.com/

Hong Kong Parkinson's Disease Foundation
http://www.hkpdf.org.hk/

Michael J. Fox Foundation for Parkinson's Research
http://www.michaeljfox.org/

National Parkinson Foundation
http://www.parkinson.org/

Northwest Parkinson's Foundation
http://www.nwpf.org/

Ohio Parkinson Foundation Northeast Region
http://www.ohparkinson.org/

Panorama Patient Network
http://www.panoramapatientnetwork.org/

Parkinson Alliance
http://www.parkinsonalliance.org/

Parkinson and Movement Disorder Alliance
http://www.pmdalliance.org/

Parkinson Association of Alberta
http://www.parkinsonalberta.ca/

Parkinson Foundation of the National Capital Area
http://www.parkinsonfoundation.org/

Parkinson Selbsthilfe Osterreich, Austria
http://www.parkinson-oesterreich.at/

Parkinson Canada
http://www.parkinson.ca/

Parkinson Study Group
http://www.parkinson-study-group.org/

Parkinson Switzerland
http://www.parkinson.ch/

Parkinson's Australia
http://www.parkinsons.org.au/

Parkinson's Disease Foundation
http://www.pdf.org/

Parkinson's Disease Society (United Kingdom) -
http://www.parkinsons.org.uk/

Parkinson's Disease Society of Slovenia
http://www.trepetlika.si/

The Parkinson's Fitness Project
https://theparkinsonsfitnessproject.com/

Parkinson's Institute and Clinical Center
http://www.thepi.org/

Parkinson's and Movement Disorder Institute
http://www.pmdi.org/

PD and Movement Disorder Society (India)
http://www.parkinsonssocietyindia.com/

Parkinson's Network
http://www.parkinsonsnetwork.org/

Parkinson's Resource Organization
http://www.parkinsonsresource.org/

Projectspark Foundation
http://www.projectspark.org/

The Cure Parkinson's Trust
http://www.cureparkinsons.org.uk/

Wisconsin Parkinson Association
http://www.wiparkinson.org/

World Parkinson Congress
http://www.worldpdcongress.org/

World Parkinson's Education Program
http://www.parkinsonseducation.org/

Online Support Groups

#nevergiveup Parkinson's and Dystonia
https://www.facebook.com/groups/325520337643000

Parkinson's Alternatives Healing
https://www.facebook.com/groups/1420381321604545

Parkinson's Community
https://www.facebook.com/groups/1301409443214325

Parkinson's Online Chat Group
https://www.facebook.com/groups/parkinsonschatroom

Young Onset PD DBS Support Forum
https://www.facebook.com/groups/dbspd

Parkinson's Journals and Newsletters

Journal of Parkinson's Disease
https://www.journalofparkinsonsdisease.com

Parkinson's Disease
https://www.hindawi.com/journals/pd/

Parkinsonism & Related Disorders
https://www.prd-journal.com

Further Reading

Books

A Parkinson's Primer by John M. Vine
https://amzn.to/2wYcH58

Parkinson's Disease: A Complete Guide by William J.
Weiner MD
https://amzn.to/2CzEkHC

Dropping the P Bomb by Emma Lawton
https://amzn.to/2wU6qam

Natural Therapies for Parkinson's Disease by Dr. Laurie
Mischley
https://amzn.to/2oSc0qe

Websites

Spoon Theory guide and resources
https://www.healthline.com/health/spoon-theory-
chronic-illness-explained-like-never-before

Clinical Trials for Parkinson's
https://www.michaeljfox.org/page.html?Participate-in-
Parkinsons-Research

Remote.co – Remote jobs
https://remote.co

Upwork – get hired as a remote freelancer or contract
worker
https://www.upwork.com

Appendix B: References

Arias-Fuenzalida, Jonathan, Javier Jarazo, Xiaobing Qing, Jonas Walter, Gemma Gomez-Giro, Sarah Louise Nickels, Holm Zaehres, Hans Robert Schöler, and Jens Christian Schwamborn. "FACS-Assisted CRISPR-Cas9 Genome Editing Facilitates Parkinson's Disease Modeling." U.S. National Library of Medicine. November 14, 2017. Accessed September 04, 2018. https://www.ncbi.nlm.nih.gov/pmc/articles/PMC5830965/.

Beal, M. Flint. "A Randomized Clinical Trial of High-Dosage Coenzyme Q10 in Early Parkinson Disease." JAMA Internal Medicine. March 24, 2014. Accessed September 04, 2018. https://jamanetwork.com/journals/jamaneurology/fullarticle/1851409.

Cohen, Jennifer. "Motivation Is A Muscle: The 7 Best Ways To Substantially Increase Your Productivity." Forbes. November 06, 2013. Accessed September 05, 2018. https://www.forbes.com/sites/jennifercohen/2013/11/06/motivation-is-a-muscle-the-7-best-ways-to-substantially-increase-your-productivity.

Dock, Elly, Elizabeth Boskey, Kathryn Watson, and Brian Wu. "Aspiration Pneumonia: Overview, Causes, and Symptoms." Healthline. August 23, 2017. Accessed September 05, 2018. https://www.healthline.com/health/aspiration-pneumonia.

Groiss, S. J., L. Wojtecki, M. Südmeyer, and A. Schnitzler. "Deep Brain Stimulation in Parkinson's Disease." U.S. National Library of Medicine. November 2009. Accessed September 04, 2018. https://www.ncbi.nlm.nih.gov/pmc/articles/PMC30 02606/.

Guttuso, Thomas, Jr., Naomi Salins, and David Lichter. "Abstract #13: Low-Dose Naltrexone's Tolerability and Effects in Fatigued Patients with Parkinson's Disease: An Open-Label Study." Egyptian Journal of Medical Human Genetics. July 17, 2010. Accessed September 04, 2018. https://www.sciencedirect.com/science/article/pii/S 1933721310000681.

"Heavy Metal Poisoning." NORD (National Organization for Rare Disorders). 2006. Accessed September 05, 2018. https://rarediseases.org/rare-diseases/heavy-metal-poisoning/.

Knekt, Paul. "High Vitamin D Levels Associated with Reduced Parkinson's Disease Risk." ScienceDaily. July 13, 2010. Accessed September 04, 2018. https://www.sciencedaily.com/releases/2010/07/100 712162624.htm.

Kocot, Joanna; Luchowska-Kocot, Dorota; Kiełczykowska, Małgorzata; Musik, Irena; Kurzepa, Jacek. 2017. "Does Vitamin C Influence Neurodegenerative Diseases and Psychiatric Disorders?" Nutrients 9, no. 7: 659.

"Medical Marijuana." Parkinson's Foundation. August 23, 2018. Accessed September 04, 2018. http://www.parkinson.org/Understanding-Parkinsons/Treatment/Medical-Marijuana.

Mo, Jia-Jie, Lin-Ying Liu, Wei-Bin Peng, Jie Rao, Zhou Liu, and Li-Li Cui. "The Effectiveness of Creatine Treatment for Parkinson's Disease: An Updated Meta-analysis of Randomized Controlled Trials." U.S. National Library of Medicine. 2017. Accessed September 04, 2018. https://www.ncbi.nlm.nih.gov/pmc/articles/PMC54 57735/.

Moldovan, Alexia-Sabine, Stefan Jun Groiss, Saskia Elben, Martin Südmeyer, Alfons Schnitzler, and Lars Wojtecki. "The Treatment of Parkinson's Disease with Deep Brain Stimulation: Current Issues." U.S. National Library of Medicine. July 2015. Accessed September 04, 2018. https://www.ncbi.nlm.nih.gov/pmc/articles/PMC45 41217/.

Mori, M. A., A. M. Delattre, B. Carabelli, C. Pudell, M. Bortolanza, P. V. Staziaki, J. V. Visentainer, P. F. Montanher, E. A. Del, and A. C. Ferraz. "Neuroprotective Effect of Omega-3 Polyunsaturated Fatty Acids in the 6-OHDA Model of Parkinson's Disease Is Mediated by a Reduction of Inducible Nitric Oxide Synthase." U.S. National Library of Medicine. June 2018. Accessed September 04, 2018. https://www.ncbi.nlm.nih.gov/pubmed/28221817.

Mythri, R. B., and M. M. Bharath. "Curcumin: A Potential Neuroprotective Agent in Parkinson's Disease." U.S. National Library of Medicine. 2012. Accessed September 04, 2018. https://www.ncbi.nlm.nih.gov/pubmed/22211691.

"Parkinson Disease - Genetics Home Reference - NIH." U.S. National Library of Medicine. May 2012. Accessed September 05, 2018.

https://ghr.nlm.nih.gov/condition/parkinson-disease#genes.

Quiroga, M J, et al. "Ascorbate- and Zinc-Responsive Parkinsonism." *U.S. National Library of Medicine.*, U.S. National Library of Medicine, Nov. 2014, www.ncbi.nlm.nih.gov/pubmed/25070397.

Sears, Barry. "A Simple Intervention in Parkinson Disease?" Medscape. May 22, 2014. Accessed September 04, 2018. https://www.medscape.com/viewarticle/825252.

Seidl, Stacey E., Jose A. Santiago, Hope Bilyk, and Judith A. Potashkin. "The Emerging Role of Nutrition in Parkinson's Disease." U.S. National Library of Medicine. March 7, 2014. Accessed September 05, 2018. https://www.ncbi.nlm.nih.gov/pmc/articles/PMC3945400/.

Sessoms, Gail. "Red Wine & Parkinson's Symptoms." LIVESTRONG.COM. October 03, 2017. Accessed September 04, 2018. http://www.livestrong.com/article/555444-red-wine-parkinsons-symptoms/.

Teesdale, Kristen. "Stem Cells Safe in Pre-Clinical Parkinson's Disease Study." The Michael J. Fox Foundation for Parkinson's Research | Parkinson's Disease. August 31, 2017. Accessed September 04, 2018. https://www.michaeljfox.org/foundation/news-detail.php?stem-cells-safe-in-pre-clinical-parkinson-disease-study.

Thiriez, Claire, Gabriel Villafane, Frédérique Grapin, Gilles Fenelon, Philippe Remy, and Pierre Cesaro. "Can Nicotine Be Used Medicinally in Parkinson's Disease?"

Medscape. 2011. Accessed September 04, 2018.
https://www.medscape.com/viewarticle/746713.

Virhammar, Johan, and Dag Nyholm. "Levodopa-carbidopa Enteral Suspension in Advanced Parkinson's Disease: Clinical Evidence and Experience." U.S. National Library of Medicine. March 2017. Accessed September 04, 2018.
https://www.ncbi.nlm.nih.gov/pmc/articles/PMC53 49373/.

Weiss, Howard D., and Laura Marsh. "Impulse Control Disorders and Compulsive Behaviors Associated with Dopaminergic Therapies in Parkinson Disease." U.S. National Library of Medicine. December 2012. Accessed September 05, 2018.
https://www.ncbi.nlm.nih.gov/pmc/articles/PMC36 13210/.

Zhao, Baolu. "Green Tea May Protect Brain Cells Against Parkinson's Disease." ScienceDaily. December 14, 2007. Accessed September 04, 2018.
https://www.sciencedaily.com/releases/2007/12/071 213101406.htm.

Zhu, Z. G., M. X. Sun, W. L. Zhang, W. W. Wang, Y. M. Jin, and C. L. Xie. "The Efficacy and Safety of Coenzyme Q10 in Parkinson's Disease: A Meta-analysis of Randomized Controlled Trials." U.S. National Library of Medicine. February 2017. Accessed September 04, 2018.
https://www.ncbi.nlm.nih.gov/pubmed/27830343.

About the Author

In 2011 Nick was diagnosed with Parkinson's disease – a disease typically affecting those over 60 – at age 33. After enduring a prolonged period of depression, he found a way to move beyond his grief and fight back by taking control of his disease, and using his experiences to educate and advocate for others. From this mission, the *Parkinson's LifeKit* app was born. The app is used by thousands of Parkinson's patients to help them take control by tracking symptoms and fitness, managing medication, and more accurately reporting on their condition to their doctors. In 2018, he launched *Parkinson's Warrior*, a Parkinson's news and resource website, which serves as a guide to adopting a Warrior Mindset to take control of each day and each battle in pursuit of improved quality of life.

In addition to being an author, app developer, and advocate, Nick is also a media studies professor. He has lived in Buenos Aires, Los Angeles, Seattle, and most recently, Amsterdam, where he lives with his wife and two cats.

Made in United States
North Haven, CT
13 November 2021

11116238R00128